Writing in English for the Medical Sciences

A PRACTICAL GUIDE

Writing in English for the Medical Sciences

A PRACTICAL GUIDE

Steve Hart
Academic Proofreader
Cambridge, England

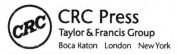

CRC Press
Taylor & Francis Group
Boca Raton   London   New York

CRC Press is an imprint of the
Taylor & Francis Group, an **informa** business

CRC Press
Taylor & Francis Group
6000 Broken Sound Parkway NW, Suite 300
Boca Raton, FL 33487-2742

© 2016 by Taylor & Francis Group, LLC
CRC Press is an imprint of Taylor & Francis Group, an Informa business

No claim to original U.S. Government works

Printed on acid-free paper
Version Date: 20151019

International Standard Book Number-13: 978-1-4987-4236-8 (Paperback)

Visit the Taylor & Francis Web site at
http://www.taylorandfrancis.com

and the CRC Press Web site at
http://www.crcpress.com

To ASEA, VDC and JH.

Contents

Preface

Academics and students in medical schools and universities worldwide are required to write in English so their work can be included in international journals and be seen by as many peers as possible. Unfortunately, a paper let down by weak English is likely to be rejected by a journal editor and the author's credibility potentially questioned; likewise, the reputation of a student will be harmed if they fail to show sufficient competence in English, regardless of their actual subject knowledge. The answer? An easily accessible resource that targets key grammar areas and that can be consulted while writing an essay or paper.

This book has been written for

Professors

Lecturers

Research officers

Graduate students

Prospective students

Industry workers

This resource has been designed to fill the gaps in the English grammar knowledge of those writers for whom English is a second or third language. It does this by providing the theory behind the language and supporting the theory by showing the actual mistakes made by students and scholars in their essays and papers. Errors made in papers authored by writers whose first language is not English are often easily fixed. The errors are either the result of gaps in knowledge or bad habits creeping in. The issue is one of awareness – and awareness can only be achieved by identifying the mistakes and then receiving instruction on how to correct them.

This book has been informed by over 300 essays and papers from the following fields:

Medicine and surgery

Cellular and molecular medicine

Immunology and infection biology

Dentistry

Nursing

Health administration

Among the features included in this book are the following:

- Fifteen chapters covering key areas of grammar and writing style
- An a–z of the terms most commonly misused by writers
- Exercises to reinforce language acquisition in key areas
- A comprehensive index of terms that can be consulted during the course of writing

The medical writer's experiences and requirements are at the heart of this resource; contrary to most guidebooks, in this resource analysis and reasoning play a supporting role to real-world examples that show the language being actively used and misused. The areas, the theory and the errors that have been included are those most relevant and, crucially, those most likely to elevate the English level of a writer to that of a native speaker. The guide's unique characteristic is this emphasis on real-world examples*. For the first time the mistakes that are actually being made in research papers and essays are addressed and directly resolved. Without them being captured and exposed, writers will continue to make them and papers will continue to be rejected and essays marked down – not because of weak research but because of weak English. My aim is to prevent this from happening to you.

Steve Hart

---

* Where necessary, examples have been modified to preserve anonymity while retaining the nature of the error.

Author

Steve Hart has been editing and proofreading for international academics and graduate students of medicine and bioscience since 2005. Formerly a high school teacher and with a background in sociolinguistics, he has written grammar guides for the Indian market and produced coursebooks for several academies in the United Kingdom. He is currently English Skills Coordinator at a higher education institution in Cambridge, England.

Complaint contents

Section I: Grammar

Complaint A: Nouns and articles

Signs: Selecting the wrong form for plural nouns, failing to recognise countable from uncountable nouns and using articles in a random way

Treatment: Fix the plurals/learn to recognise uncountable nouns/ realise that some nouns can be both/comprehend compounds/ understand the definite article/understand the indefinite and zero articles/grasp proper nouns and fixed phrases/appreciate when the article can be omitted/recognise the common errors

Complaint B: Verbs

Signs: Getting the forms of 'to be' mixed up, using the wrong verb ending, failing to match the subject and the verb, not adapting to the addition of a modal

Treatment: Study the verb 'to be'/ensure the subject agrees with the verb/realise that some verb forms are not really verbs/meet with the modals/appreciate the abstract nature of phrasal verbs

Complaint C: Adjectives and adverbs

Signs: Inability to choose between adjectives and adverbs, problems with choosing a suitable description and failing to realise which quantifiers take singular and plural nouns and verbs

Treatment: Recognise the lack of relationship between certain adjectives and adverbs/learn the endings/put the adverb in its place/know how to compare/get past the past participle/Are your adjectives excessive?/compare specific terms/recognise other errors/learn which quantifiers are singular or plural/recognise the meaning of the 'of' phrase/ note the errors

Complaint D: Prepositions

Signs: Finding it difficult to choose among the prepositions

Treatment: Learn the prepositional relationships and common phrases

Complaint E: Clauses

Signs: Failing to appreciate dependent clauses, using the wrong connecting words, creating sentences with the wrong construction

Treatment: Recognise the clause categories/select the correct conjunction/understand the conditions/recognise the errors

Complaint F: Prefixes

Signs: Inability to interpret the meaning of unfamiliar terms, failing to select the correct prefix

Treatment: Recognise the correct form/know when to use hyphens

Section II: Elements and data

Complaint G: Time

Signs: Confusing prepositions, not knowing when to use the singular form, failing to use the correct tense

Treatment: Select the correct prep/learn when to keep things singular/learn key time phrases/keep to the right tense/eradicate certain errors

Complaint H: People

Signs: Using unsuitable terms for patients, ages and races

Treatment: Learn which terms to use

Complaint I: Numbers and stats

Signs: Misusing numbers and percentages, confusing statistical terms

Treatment: Learn a few conventions/organise the units of measure/know where to position the number/use percentages correctly/recognise when to use rank/work with ranges/note the common mistakes/check the stats

Section III: Style

Complaint J: Tense

Signs: Having trouble forming tenses, inability to select the correct tense

Treatment: Learn the aspects/know when to change tenses/plan for the future

Complaint K: Verbs and voice

Signs: Failing to understand the relationship between active and passive writing, using weak verb forms, using the wrong verbs for reporting and claiming

Treatment: Understand the relationship between voice and tense/ appreciate the merits of both voices/be aware of nominalisation/ understand that verbs can take on strong and weak properties/know which verbs should be used for claims/know which verbs should be used for reporting

Complaint L: Clarity and character

Signs: Writing inefficiently and without focus, using the wrong style and vocabulary

Treatment: Avoid redundant and unnecessary terms/make sure to prioritise the subject/eliminate most conjunctions/keep the verbs parallel/retain the abstract style/move some data to tables

Complaint M: Spelling and punctuation

Signs: Misspelling terms and using the wrong punctuation

Treatment: Be aware of the most commonly misspelled words/know the differences between AE and BE/master apostrophe use/distinguish the dashes/be conscious of the comma/limit the capitals/place the parentheses

Complaint N: Titles

Signs: Using a title that is irrelevant and unhelpful

Treatment: Select a title that suits your paper

Complaint O: References

Signs: Failing to cite correctly in the main text, creating an unsatisfactory reference list

Treatment: Utilise the number system/know what to look for/ eliminate agreement and grammar errors

SECTION I

Grammar

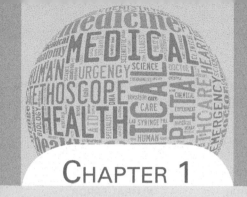

CHAPTER 1

Complaint A: Nouns and articles

> Signs:
> → Selecting the wrong form for plural nouns
> → Failing to recognise countable from uncountable nouns
> → Using articles in a random way

Nouns

Treatment

In order to use nouns correctly an understanding of the concept of boundedness is required. Boundedness tells us whether a noun can be counted or not and therefore whether a plural can be formed. The concept is helpful in explaining why some nouns can be both countable and uncountable. To know if a noun can be counted we need to work out whether it has a clear 'boundary' and can be seen as a clearly separate thing, either physically or in our minds. In other words, does it have a clear beginning and end?

Cigarette – The noun 'cigarette' is a separate entity that can be counted.

*They looked at the number of **cigarettes** smoked in a week…*

Fix the plurals

Once a noun has been identified as countable the next step is to learn how to form the plural. Many plural nouns end in 's' or 'es' but there are a few different variations.

Keep an eye on these plurals as they are troublesome:

SINGULAR	PLURAL	PLURAL ERROR
analysis (see also a–z)	**analyses**	analysis
axis	**axes**	axi/axises
bacillus	**bacilli**	bacilles
biopsy	**biopsies**	biopsys
cannula	**cannulae/cannulas**	cannuli
chorda	**chordae**	chordas
cortex	**cortices**	cortexes
diagnosis (see also a–z)	**diagnoses**	diagnosis
fibula	**fibulae/fibulas**	fibuli
gyrus	**gyri**	gyruses
hypothesis	**hypotheses**	hypothesis
index	**indexes/indices**[a]	indexs
intermediary	**intermediaries**	intermediares
lamina	**laminae**	laminas
metastasis	**metastases**	metastes
ovum	**ova**	ovums
paralysis	**paralyses**	paralysis
prosthesis (see also a–z)	**prostheses**	prosthetics
remedy	**remedies**	remedys
sequela	**sequelae**	sequels
stimulus	**stimuli**	stimulises/stimulis
varix	**varices**	varicies

[a] Usually financial.

> **CASE REPORT: BACTERIA/COHORT/CRITERIA/DATA**
>
> **Case 1: Bacteria**   Bacterium is the singular form and bacteria is the plural.
>
> *Some of the intestinal bacteria ~~was~~ **(were)** inhibited by this process.*
>
> *This **bacterium** is different in the way it forms its growth chains.*
>
> **Case 2: Cohort**   In the medical sciences, cohort is used to refer to a group and therefore is considered singular. The plural 'cohorts' can refer to groups or to individuals within a cohort but the singular form is by far the most common use of the noun.
>
> *A **cohort** of 3000 patients treated with low-intensity pulsed ultrasound was...*
>
> **Case 3: Criteria**   This is a plural noun. The singular is criterion.
>
> *The **criterion was** width greater than 40% of depth.*
>
> *The **criteria were** width greater than 40% of depth, frequency at 15 dB...*
>
> **Case 4: Data**   Although used with a singular and a plural verb, it is common practice to treat data as a plural. The singular 'datum' is infrequently used. Data also has uncountable properties so cannot be used with numbers (~~three data~~) or quantity words used with plurals (both, few, many, several...)
>
> *There is much data on the long-term effects of this...*

Learn to recognise uncountable nouns

Nouns that cannot be counted do not have clear boundaries. They have no clear parts that can be separated or enclosed. They are all part of the whole without any obvious limits. These uncountable nouns are usually concepts, processes, ideas, qualities, substances or emotions.

Help – uncountable

*I would also like to acknowledge the participating elderly residents for their **help** in providing useful information...*

It is important to remember that an uncountable noun cannot have an indefinite article (a/an) in front of it.

~~A~~ help from the cardiology team allowed us to...

It also cannot have a plural form.

*They have been kind enough to extend their ~~helps~~ (**help**) at various stages of the trial.*

Here are a few more uncountable nouns to be aware of:

access	help	reliability
advice (see also a–z)	information	research
assistance	knowledge	safety
caution	literature	staff
consent	management	support
coverage	patience	training
equipment	potential	thirst
evidence	progress	trust

The confusing thing is that some nouns can be both countable and uncountable. It all depends on the way the noun is being used by the writer and the context.

*The treatment plan was initially drawn up on **paper**.*

*I had a number of **papers** that needed to be submitted before the end of term.*

The first example of the noun 'paper' is referring to the substance and is therefore uncountable. But in the second example the writer is referring to specific essay papers which can naturally be counted (they have a number of them).

Nouns that can be both countable and uncountable are often countable when the writer is referring to a specific instance or kind; they are uncountable when a general concept or sense is intended. Some take on different meanings in their countable and uncountable forms (e.g. ground/grounds).

absence	evaluation	prediction
achievement	experience	pressure
assessment	ground	protection
behaviour	growth	society
classification	industry	strategy
communication	influence	strength
concern (see also a–z)	investigation	success (see also a–z)

context	language	teaching
control	level	technology
degree	light	theory
development	performance	thought
disease	perspective (see also a–z)	time
effect (see also a–z)	policy	understanding
environment	power	work

Experience plays a large part in being able to assess the accuracy of the patient's account.

*We then surveyed the **experiences** of the nurses working at this unit.*

– communication

Communication is a good example of a noun that writers frequently use in a countable way when the uncountable form would be more appropriate. Unless a particular act of communication is being referred to, the writer is likely to require the uncountable form with a zero article to signify a general meaning.

~~Communications are~~ (***Communication is***) *vital between a patient and their carer.*

CASE REPORT: OBSESSIVE COUNTABILITY

As alluded to above, when faced with a choice many writers will use a plural when actually the uncountable (concept) form would be more suitable. When the uncountable form is required, the context will relate to theory rather than to events.

The plural form is also mistakenly used for uncountable nouns that have no countable form, which is clearly a more severe error.

They offer general ~~advices~~ on exercise, fatigue ~~managements~~ and other matters relating to health ~~educations~~.

Comprehend compounds

Nouns that are made up of two or more parts are called compounds. Some are written as one word and should not be split up.

background   baseline
benchmark   bypass (see also a–z)
endpoint   intake (see also a–z)
lifetime   offset
onset   outcome
outbreak   outset

> ...in combination with reduced fluid ~~in-take~~ (**intake**). Future research should focus on clinical ~~end-points~~ (**endpoints**)...

Others can be split up to become phrasal verbs (pv).

cutoff (noun) – a limit or point of termination

cut off (pv) – to separate or isolate; to stop suddenly or shut off

feedback (noun) – the return of information; a response within a system

feed back (pv) – to submit information

followup (noun) – a subsequent examination to assess earlier treatment

follow up (pv) – to increase success by further action

Other compounds are formed from combinations of nouns, adjectives, verbs or prepositions but they are always treated as a single unit.

*Identifying issues concerning **patient data** is a key objective...*

When the term consists of more than one word, the initial word(s) acts like an adjective (it may even be an adjective) and modifies the final word. When the first word is a noun like in this next example, the temptation is to use the plural form.

*~~Autoantibodies~~ (**Autoantibody**) detection is a useful investigative method that can...*

↑

Autoantibody detection is a compound term made up of two nouns. The first word of a compound should be in singular form, unless it is one of those terms that modifies as a plural, e.g. customs/systems/earnings (as seen in systems analyst and earnings forecast). Most compounds have a generic, uncountable meaning rather than detailing an actual situation.

An alternative in some situations is to use 'Detection of autoantibodies'. Note how the plural is acceptable in the 'of phrase' but not in the compound noun.

Here are two more examples where the modifying terms need to be singular.

A stem ~~cells~~ (cell) transplant from the bone marrow shows...

This was a clinical presentation of the disease in the ~~adults~~ (adult) population.

Some terms cannot make compounds and instead are written as 'of phrases'.

It is the fourth most common ~~death cause~~ (cause of death)....

They looked at the endocardial ~~origin sites~~ (sites of origin)...

She was also experiencing ~~breath shortness~~ (shortness of breath).

INTERVENTION   **plural phrases**

For plural phrases, the first word is plural but the second is singular.

levels of intensity   level of ~~intensities~~
schools of thought   school of ~~thoughts~~

Here the 'of phrase' is not an option and the compound must be used.

When this happens ~~the success of treatment~~ (treatment success) is limited.

If in doubt search for the particular pattern of words to see how they can be linked as a phrase.

– separate the nouns from the verbs

Confusing nouns with verbs is a common fault in medical papers. Nouns have many endings but a number of them end in –sion and –tion; remembering this should help with combating the verb/noun problem.

This will aid the ~~detect~~ (detection) of breast cancer... (see also a–z)

Nouns are in bold (see also a–z entries)

averse	**aversion**	compress	**compression**
confuse	**confusion**	consult	**consultation**
consume	**consumption**	distribute	**distribution**
exclude	**exclusion**	expect	**expectation**
intervene	**intervention**	obstruct	**obstruction**
reduce	**reduction**	regulate	**regulation**
resume	**resumption**	stimulate	**stimulation**

Articles

Treatment

An article is a word that is used before a noun to indicate the kind of reference being made to the noun.

definite article = *the*   indefinite article = *a/an*

zero article = no article used

Articles in English help the reader to identify and follow the nouns in a sentence and to understand the relationship between them and the other parts of the sentence. The terms in bold are where the writer has had to make an article decision for the noun 'study':

Dissolution studies are not able to predict this performance effectively. For instance, a study demonstrating the results of in vitro dissolution tests failed to provide satisfactory correlations. The study was carried out...

A recent study has shown that this correlates best with the in vivo percentage absorbed data (43). Unfortunately, the study of drug development has been complicated by unnecessary...

In these two paragraphs there are two definite articles, two indefinite articles and a zero article connected with the noun 'study'. However, only one article decision has been influenced by another instance of the noun in the passage. Can you work out which one?

'The study was carried out' was the only time the article choice ('the') was influenced by another instance of 'study'.

Understand the definite article

If the writer can single out a noun as unique from the context of the sentence, and if the reader will be able to understand the exact thing being described, then the noun can take a definite article.

So, for a noun to be definite the reader must be aware of the exact thing the writer is referring to.

> *There are three structures in the red cell membrane: **a lipid bilayer**, membrane proteins embedded into **the lipid bilayer**, and...*

The definite article is used here because the writer has introduced the lipid bilayer so the reader can follow the reference.

Therefore, one way a noun can be definite is if it has already been mentioned. A second way that a noun can be definite is the reader having prior knowledge of the noun because of a logical situation.

> *A research study looked at the management of orofacial granulomatosis. **The researcher's** approach was to...*

Here, the researcher had not been previously mentioned but the reader should be aware that a research study is carried out by a researcher. The reader can make an association between the two nouns and therefore the writer uses 'the'.

The reader can also be made aware of the definiteness of the noun if the phrase following it creates a direct association based on the physical surroundings.

***The administrators in the clinic** did not have a system in place to log this information.*

Similarly, the definite sense can be used in this next example because the reader will again understand the context. The reader will know that the clock being referred to is in the room where the presentation took place.

*After we presented the findings of our study, we looked at **the clock** and realised we had spoken for over twenty five minutes.*

The writer can also use a definite article when referring to somebody or something that there can only be one of. This is apparent in terms like *most, best, least and last*. These terms exclude all other things and leave just one – so logically the reader will understand that the noun is definite, that only one is being referred to and which one that is.

*Measurement of the phenolic acid formation appeared to be **the best** option...*

The definite article can also be used when a singular noun represents its entire type in a general sense. The noun stands as an example of its type (like a prototype) and a general statement is made about this type as a whole.

> ***The practitioner** should be more aware of the dynamics affecting the strategy.*

> Here, the practitioner is being used to represent all practitioners. The writer is not referring to a specific one but practitioners as a whole.

So the awareness of the reader can allow the writer to give nouns definite articles. But the writer must also ensure that the noun is able to be singled out for definiteness from the context of the sentence.

Changing this procedure also had ~~the~~ significant effect on the results.

Here, the writer cannot single out 'significant effect' as unique and definite because it is not the only significant effect and this is additional information that the writer is simply using in a general way. The indefinite article (*a*) is required instead.

*Changing this procedure also had **a** significant effect on the results.*

Understand the indefinite and zero articles

A noun is used in an indefinite way when the writer either knows the reader will not be aware of the exact thing being mentioned or does not require the reader to know.

*A **hospital** in Glasgow was the setting for the pilot. Stobhill Hospital was chosen because...*

In the sentence above the writer has yet to introduce the hospital to the reader so the noun has taken an indefinite article. They then go on to name the hospital in the next sentence.

> *There is a specialised cardiology unit at L_____and also at a **clinic** to the north of the city.*
> ↑
>> In this sentence the writer has mentioned a clinic in the city but only to make the reader aware that there is another place offering cardiac care. The reader is unlikely to know this clinic and the writer has no intention of mentioning it again or providing further details.

In indefinite situations, if the noun is singular and countable an indefinite article ('a/an') should be used. If it is uncountable or plural then a zero article (no article) is used.

> *They are hoping for more **government support** and also **funding** from **private investors**.* ↑
>> The exact type or kind of funding and support and who these investors are have yet to be identified. So the writer uses zero articles for the three instances and they have the equivalent meaning of 'some'.

The zero article can also be substituted for 'some' in the following example:

*But there will be (some) **compounds** that are not absorbed.*

The noun is also indefinite when it is being used as an example of its kind or type. The writer here is being generic and uses a singular countable noun:

*A **hospital manager** needs to adapt to these changing needs.*

If a plural noun is used to achieve this then a zero article will be required.

***Hospital managers** have greater financial constraints than private sector bosses...*

—Realise specific does not necessarily mean definite

These last examples were generic, but it is important to understand that the noun can be indefinite even if the writer is using it in a specific sense. It is only ever definite if the reader has exact knowledge of the particular one or thing. This was seen in the earlier example '...*also at a clinic to the north of the city'*. The clinic exists (it is a specific clinic) but it has not been identified and the reader does not have sufficient information.

specific

*There was **a patient** who withdrew during the second stage.*

indefinite

It is not important here to identify the patient who left; the reader just needs to be informed that someone withdrew during stage two. This is also true when discussing conditions and diseases. They are specific illnesses but have an indefinite and generic meaning when they are being referred to and therefore usually take a zero article.

~~The~~ *oesophageal cancer can develop without showing any symptoms...*

INTERVENTION   **such**

When using such to mean 'this type of', make sure an indefinite article is used before a singular countable noun.

Such (a) problem can be managed by following a specific routine...

CASE REPORT: TYPE A OR TYPE AN?

Use 'a' when the noun following has a consonant sound when it is spoken.

a treatment   a diet   a placebo

Use 'an' when the noun following has a vowel sound when it is spoken.

an inhibitory effect   an assessment

If a noun beginning with 'h' is spoken softly like an 'o' then use 'an'.

an hour   an honest error

If a noun beginning with 'eu' or 'u' has a 'you' sound then use 'a'.

a European study   a unique approach

If a noun beginning with 'o' has a 'wa' sound then 'a' is used.

a one-to-one session

For numbers, remember to think of how it is spelled when written.

An 8-week control (eight)   *An 11 mm incision* (eleven)

Also for abbreviations, think about the sound of the first letter.

an STI (S = es)   *a PAHBAH solution   an MRI scan* (M = em)

Remember that the word immediately after the indefinite article will indicate whether you use 'a' or 'an.'

A sequence of housekeeping genes   An additional sequence of...

– identify the options available (countable)

Every time a writer encounters a noun or noun phrase they must select an article to use. If we take the noun 'colony' and assume the writer has recognised its countability, then there are several options.

- A definite article (*the colony*)
- An indefinite article (*a colony*)
- Plural form with a zero article (*colonies*)
- Plural form with a definite article (*the colonies*)
- Another determiner word (*this colony/each colony...*)

> 'Colony' in the singular form can only take a zero article if it is part of a name or compound.
>
> *Colony 2 has grown between...*
>
> *The effect of colony variation is...*

The only option the writer does not have and the one they often choose is a zero article with the singular form.

This was prior to colony being inoculated in...   ✗

– recognising uncountable nouns

When uncountable nouns are modified by an adjective it may be harder to remember not to use a/an.

There is a clear evidence for why the levels did not rise...

> Why did the writer make this mistake?
>
> Earlier in the paragraph the writer had written 'there is a clear difference between...' As difference is countable this is fine. Perhaps they were influenced by the adjective and began with 'a clear...' again without considering whether the noun following was countable (in this case 'evidence' – uncountable); or perhaps they were unaware that evidence was uncountable.

Grasp proper nouns and fixed phrases

A proper noun is different from a typical or common noun in that it states the actual name of the person, place or thing.

Common noun: *person*   Common noun: *clinic*

Proper noun: **Dr Samuels**   Proper noun: **Redlands**

Although they have a definite sense, proper nouns will usually take a zero article.

We would like to thank ~~the~~ Kulzer & Co and ~~the~~ Dr Azman Reno for their materials and valuable input respectively.

However, proper nouns take a definite article if 'the' is seen as part of their name or common usage has led them to take 'the'.

*We will now compare the rates in **the United Kingdom** and Hong Kong.*

Fixed phrases are phrases that are in general use and are familiar to native speakers. Some of these phrases do not contain a definite article even though they have a definite sense. The meaning may also be different to what would be expected; in essence, looking at the literal meaning of each individual word may not reveal the true meaning of the phrase.

*The patients' records were also **out of date**.* ~~out of the date~~

*This has been covered **at length**.* ~~at a length~~

*The findings will certainly be **of interest**.* ~~of their interest~~

– example errors

at first	at ~~the~~ first	**at present**	at ~~the~~ present
in advance	in ~~an~~ advance	**in place**	in ~~the~~ place
in practice	in ~~the~~ practice	**in private**	in ~~the~~ private
in turn	in ~~a~~ turn	**area of interest**	area of ~~an~~ interest
on purpose	on ~~the~~ purpose	**on/in time**	in ~~a~~ time

***At present**, few studies have investigated this deficiency...*

*A pilot was performed **in advance** so as to understand...*

Here is a pair of fixed phrases where the definite article completely changes the meaning of the phrase:

In the case – regarding   In case – if it should happen

*A tube can be inserted **in case** the bleeding cannot be stopped.*

*This might not be completely true **in the case** of obesity.*

Appreciate when the article can be omitted

As scientists often look to describe general principles and processes, the definite article is disregarded at times in scientific papers.

***Testing of this drug** was done over the course of one week.*

Things being tested are often stripped of their definite status and made generic, despite unique events being described. This is especially true of plural nouns.

***Outcomes** were based on **movements** carried out and **problems** encountered during the trial.*

This style (although concise) will sound imprecise, become tedious and eventually prove ambiguous for the reader if employed throughout the text. An article can add precision and aid understanding – and in some cases be essential to the meaning. Indeed, those who judge articles to be largely unnecessary and believe better clarity can be achieved by striking out every single one should examine the following robotic extract:

> *Post-mortem study found that long term treatment with anticholinergic drugs can promote formation of senile plaque in brain. Earlier study showed that balance between dopamine and acetylcholine level regulating signal in striatum is primary reason for...*

Recognise the common errors

An overall improvements in function has been reported (12).

> Plurals are often mistakenly used with indefinite articles and vice versa.

This resulted in reduced clotting and a serious bleeding episodes.

> *Various studies have shown this to be an (a) useful tool for early detection and a (an) OHC analysis has revealed that...*

> Remember the rules around when to use a and when to use an.

These drugs will be metabolised in (the) liver.

> *Liver enzyme metabolism is the final biochemical parameter.*

> Parts of the body usually require a definite article unless they are modifying another noun.

Patients suspected of suffering from the bulimia nervosa...

> *A Plummer–Vinson syndrome is characterised by a...*
> *The oesophageal cancer is becoming increasingly common...*

> Most conditions, diseases and ailments take the zero article.

*~~The~~ supersaturation in intestinal fluid is ~~the~~ **(an)** important property that can play ~~the~~ **(a)** significant role in ~~the~~ drug absorption.* ↑

> Overuse of the definite article can be caused by a failure to appreciate when a noun is a unique instance and when it is being used in general terms or as an example.

*~~Authors~~ **(The authors)** gratefully acknowledge ___ for partially funding this research.*

*(**A**) resistance exercise was introduced at week 3.* ↑

> An uncountable noun can be used to modify another noun. Here the indefinite article is used before the uncountable noun but it is referring to the countable noun 'exercise' and not the uncountable 'resistance'.

Chapters, figures...

A definite article will often be used when referring to a chapter, figure, equation, etc.

*In **the next chapter** we will evaluate the different...*

The determiner 'this' can also be employed.

*In **this chapter** the process will be investigated...*

But when writing the number of the chapter, figure or equation it is effectively being named and so changes to a proper noun with a zero article.

~~The~~ Figure 3 below shows the relationship between the two...

With next, previous, following, etc. a number is unnecessary.

This will be shown in the following chapter ~~6~~.

In the next chapter ~~5~~ we address...

CASE REPORT: DISTRACTIONS

Often a noun will have information attached to it that modifies it in some way. Usually it is an adjective or another noun. The writer may forget to use an article with the original noun because the article is not directly next to the noun and the descriptive word or phrase creates a distraction.

*This will be **a lengthy and complex treatment** that is likely to…*

The article here is relating to the noun 'treatment' which is a few words along.

0.7 and 0.75 are regarded as ~~an~~ acceptable test reliability scores.

The article here is relating to the noun 'scores' which is a few words along, but the plural cannot take an indefinite article.

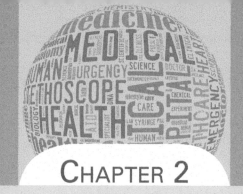

CHAPTER 2

Complaint B: Verbs

Signs:
- → Confusing forms of the verb 'to be'
- → Failing to match the verb with the subject
- → Experiencing verbal problems
- → Misusing modals
- → Not recognising phrasal verb meanings

Treatment

The verb 'to be' is everywhere. It is difficult to write a paragraph without at least one or two forms of the verb making an appearance. As well as being the most common verb it is also the most difficult to understand. Realising which form to use with each tense and with other auxiliaries and mastering 'being', 'been' and 'has been' are the areas on which to focus.

To be

1. To take place; to occur
2. To exist or live

Present participle: **being**   Past participle: **been**

PAST

Simple		Perfect	
I	was	I	had been
he/she	was	he/she	had been
it	was	it	had been
we/they	were	we/they	had been

Progressive		Perfect progressive	
I	was being	I	had been being
he/she	was being	he/she	had been being
it	was being	it	had been being
we/they	were being	we/they	had been being

PRESENT

Simple		Perfect	
I	am	I	have been
he/she	is	he/she	has been
it	is	it	has been
we/they	are	we/they	have been

Progressive		Perfect progressive	
I	am being	I	have been being
he/she	is being	he/she	has been being
it	is being	it	has been being
we/they	are being	we/they	have been being

FUTURE

Simple		Perfect	
I	will be	I	will have been
he/she	will be	he/she	will have been
it	will be	it	will have been
we/they	will be	we/they	will have been

Progressive		Perfect progressive	
I	will be being	I	will have been being
he/she	will be being	he/she	will have been being
it	will be being	it	will have been being
we/they	will be being	we/they	will have been being

– when to use 'been' and 'being'

The verb form 'being' is the present participle of the verb and is used for the present progressive tense.

We will now look at how they are ~~been~~ *(**being**) affected.*

The form 'been' is the past participle. Unlike most participles, these two forms cannot be used as adjectives.

> Sometimes 'being' and 'been' are confused but from the list above it is clear that 'been' is always found after the verb 'to have'.

have been

A series of clinical trials ~~been~~ *conducted to examine…*

been

These compounds have ~~being~~ *associated with anticarcinogenic and antioxidant properties.*

Errors also occur when the sentence includes

– despite   – as well as/also   – due to

The simple form of the verb (is/are/was/were) cannot be used in the following sentences, they require 'being'.

being

Despite these results ~~are~~ *rather mixed, we can still draw a few conclusions.*

being

As well as ~~was~~ *intrusive, it also has a poor success rate.*

Being

~~Been~~ *involved in this project has given me the opportunity to increase my knowledge.*

It is useful to remember that 'being' is the form to use after a preposition.

*Those in the field insist **on being** cautious about claiming…*

– when to use 'has been' and 'was'

Looking at the list in the introduction we can see that 'was' is the simple past form of the verb and 'has been' is the present perfect.

So 'was' is used to describe something that happened in the past and has now finished.

*'I didn't feel that it **was** doing a lot of good at the time'*

'has been' is used to describe something that happened in the past but the actual time of the event is not important. It may be linked with something continuing today. There is some overlap between 'was' and 'has been' but the error is made when a particular point in time is used. A particular point in time usually means that the present perfect (*has been*) cannot be used.

*In 2000 a new strategy ~~has been~~ (**was**) announced with the aim of targeting specific areas of healthcare.*

But 'has been' is used along with 'since' for a point in time if the event is still continuing today.

*The spokesperson for the local carer groups (who since 2011 ~~was~~ (**has been**) Mr D___) was also present.*

Remember to include the 'been' part:

Many results have obtained for this particular subgroup.   ✗

Several types of antibiotics have successfully used to treat symptoms.   ✗

Ensure the subject agrees with the verb

The main purpose of the three group discussions were to understand why they made those treatment choices. ✗	The main purpose of the three group discussions was to understand why they made those treatment choices. ✓

In order to make the verb agree with the subject in a sentence, ask three questions:

What is the **subject** of the sentence?	*The **main purpose** of the three…*
Is the subject singular or plural?	singular (*main purpose*)
Does the verb match the subject?	*was* (singular) YES

Making the subject agree with the verb is not a straightforward procedure. Here are some useful pointers to make the task easier.

To ensure that you select the correct verb form you must identify the subject. The subject will be a person or place, idea or thing that is doing something or being something.

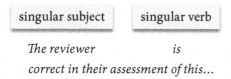

| singular subject | singular verb |

The reviewer   is
correct in their assessment of this…

– sometimes it is not easy to identify the subject
There may be a singular or plural noun in the sentence causing confusion. If it is not the subject it should not affect the verb form.

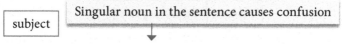

*The **role** of the carers ~~are~~ **(is)** crucial here.*

Similarly with a singular noun,

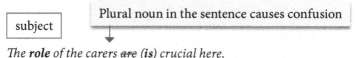

*The **amplitudes** in the **tinnitus group** ~~was~~ **(were)** compared
with those from…*

The subject normally comes before the verb, but with sentences that are questions or begin with 'There' or 'It is' the verb can be found before the subject.

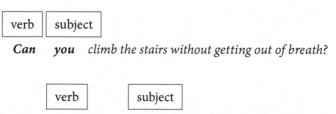

| verb | subject |

Can   you   *climb the stairs without getting out of breath?*

| verb | | subject |

*There **were** three **possible reasons** for the inflammation:*

The subject may be a verbal ending in –ing.

> subject

***Sequencing** of the whole exome can also be carried out.*

The subject may also be 'it' referring to a later expression.

> subject ——————   (see also a–z *it*)

It** was apparent **that the problem originated elsewhere.

– avoid two subjects

Check that the subject has not been repeated in the sentence. Here a pronoun has been added unnecessarily.

subject	subject repeated

The **study** ~~it~~ has the advantage of testing three different specimens.

subject	subject repeated

...and the **oxygen levels** ~~they~~ *were increased by shaking bacterial cultures.*

– know which form to choose

The presence of antibodies in the plasma | was/were | *determined by the agglutination process.*

> In this instance 'presence' is the key phrase (not 'antibodies') so the singular form **'was'** is used.

The method used for determining those segments  *the $2^{-\Delta Ct}$ method.*

In this instance 'method' is the key phrase (not 'segments') so the singular form '**is**' is used.

Thus, looking for suitable subjects 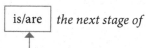 *the next stage of the process.*

In this instance 'looking' is the key phrase (not 'subjects') so the singular form '**is**' is used.

ASSESSMENT   **quantity**

When using phrases that indicate portions or quantity (majority, percentage, some...), the noun after 'of' will determine whether to use a singular or plural verb.

A third of the fibre is from this source. (fibre = singular)

A third of all deaths were from CVD. (deaths = plural)

– when using collective nouns...

Groups of people are often considered a single unit and therefore take a singular verb.

*The active group ~~were~~ (**was**) given four different...*

But groups can also be thought of as containing a number of individuals, and when certain individuals within the group are being referred to or part of the group has different characteristics or views then the noun can take a plural verb.

*The active group **were** changing their minds about this as well.*
(Perhaps not all but some at least)

When single quantifiers or determiners are used, the verb must be singular.

*Each group ~~were~~ (**was**) allocated a set period in which...* (see Complaint C)

– when faced with two uncountable nouns...
If the two nouns are separated by 'and', then use a plural verb form.

- uncountable AND uncountable = plural

  *Fruit and vegetables **are** recommended for all...*

- uncountable OR uncountable = singular

  *Pain or discomfort **is** usually experienced in the...*

However, some nouns together are considered a single entity and therefore take the singular verb form.

*Research and development **is** a crucial factor in this.*

– some more subject/verb examples

> *Personalised medicine, to treat sight-threatening conditions, ~~are~~ (**is**) an outcome of the technological advances made...*

> Clauses between commas can serve as a distraction and should have no effect on the singular/plural verb choice.

*The risks ~~increases~~ (**increase**) with age and also...*

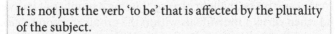

> It is not just the verb 'to be' that is affected by the plurality of the subject.

Realise that some verb forms are not really verbs
Verbals represent a challenging area for the writer of English in that although they are derived from verbs, they actually function as nouns, adjectives or adverbs in a sentence.

Three types are recognised:

Gerunds – ***Comparing*** *the cell lines to their original source led us to the identification of these genes.*

These verb forms end in –ing and act like nouns.

Participles – *This is said to play a key role in the **developing** nervous system.*

These verb forms usually end in –ing or –ed and act like adjectives.

Infinitives – *We randomised them **to investigate** the effect on satiety and body weight.*

These verb forms are usually preceded by 'to' and act like nouns, adjectives or adverbs.

– when to use the –ing form

It is useful to recognise the three different forms in your writing but the dilemma at the practical level is usually whether to use the 'to' form or the –ing form. It can depend on the verb that precedes the verbal. Some verbs will only be followed by the –ing form, whereas others may require the 'to' form.

The verb 'to suggest' will always be followed by –ing:

The authors suggest to assess the intervention types by using a checklist that contains...   ✗

*The authors **suggest assessing** the intervention types by using a checklist that contains...*   ✓

Other verbs that are followed by the –ing form include avoid, consider, delay, finish, keep, postpone, recommend, require, risk.

*We delayed **administering** this drug for two hours.*

*The organisation has recommended **using** a standardized system to describe each bony segment.*

A useful rule to remember is that the –ing form must always be used after a preposition.

*A more comprehensive approach paved the way for **reaching** a final diagnosis.*

– understand present and past participles

There are two kinds of participle, the present and the past. The present participle always ends in –ing.

*We are looking to reduce the **processing** time.*

The past participle ends in –ed for regular verbs but has various endings for irregular verbs.

*The **published** data demonstrates widespread clinical studies on the impacts of GHD.*

*The **written** accounts must be analysed before we can…*

These participles also help to form the present and progressive tenses. The wrong participle might be selected either because of the active/passive nature of the sentence or because it lacks a relationship with the noun it is modifying.

*The changed (**changing**) pattern of the virus is a concern…*

*We will also address the underlined (**underlying**) mechanisms that…*

The present participle usually has an active meaning and the past participle a passive meaning. But there are some past participles that can produce an active phrase.

*This is an **advanced** method for dealing with the issue.*

Writers should also consider the following areas of difficulty.

Simple past and past participle

The past participle is used after the verb 'to have' to form the perfect tense and for passive constructions. If the verb is an irregular verb it will have a different past participle form to the past tense form. arise – irregular verb (see also a–z *rise*)

*The idea **arose** from observing motility patterns…*   simple past tense

*The hip was being treated but the initial problem had **arisen** in the lower back.*   past perfect tense / past participle form is used

It is a common error to use the simple past for an irregular verb in the perfect tense or in a passive sentence.

*For this project, compounds CA, CS and CX were chose (**chosen**).*

CASE REPORT: BEGIN/CHOOSE/SEEK/TAKE/UNDERGO/WITHDRAW

These six irregular cases cause problems when the past participle is required. Note the following forms and examples.

Case 1: **Begin**

simple present	begin
simple past	began
past participle	begun
present participle	beginning

*Their symptoms had ~~began~~ (**begun**) not more than 12 months before...*

Case 2: **Choose**

simple present	choose
simple past	chose
past participle	chosen
present participle	choosing

*The criteria for ~~chosing~~ (**choosing**) appropriate predesigned TGEA pairs are as follows:*

Case 3: **Seek**

simple present	seek
simple past	sought
past participle	sought
present participle	seeking

*After that we ~~seeked~~ (**sought**) to identify which family members were involved for each cell type.*

Case 4: **Take**

simple present	take
simple past	took
past participle	taken
present participle	taking

*These bioactivities were not ~~took~~ (**taken**) into consideration.*

Case 5: **Undergo**

simple present	undergo
simple past	underwent
past participle	undergone
present participle	undergoing

*Participants of the studies were out-patients that had ~~underwent~~ (**undergone**) colonoscopy.*

Case 6: **Withdraw**

	simple present	withdraw
	simple past	withdrew
	past participle	withdrawn
	present participle	withdrawing

*One of the specimens was ~~withdrew~~ (**withdrawn**) from the study.*

– avoid modifiers that dangle

As well as a single participle modifying a noun as seen above, verbals can also be found in phrases that collectively modify the noun.

Examining this possibility, *the unit prepared three interventions for group two.*

The phrase is modifying the subject (*the unit*) and appears directly before it. A common error is to create a dangling modifier whereby the phrase has no obvious subject attached to it or it modifies the wrong subject.

Addressing these issues, the trial moved to a weekend...   ✗

Addressing these issues, we moved the trial to a weekend...   ✓

The dangling modifier in the first example creates the impression that the trial instigated the move.

– know when to use the infinitive

The verb 'to expect' will always be followed by the infinitive form. (see also a–z *expect*)

We expect ~~seeing~~ an improvement within a few hours.   ✗

*We expect **to see** an improvement within a few hours.*   ✓

Other verbs that are followed by the infinitive include agree, attempt, decide, intend, learn, need, plan, propose, want.

We need to extend these studies using molecular methods.

An individual might decide to quit smoking after being influenced by...

Some verbs can be followed by the infinitive form or the –ing form with little or no change in meaning: begin, continue, like, prefer, remember, start, try.

*Cells will continue **to grow/growing** until they synthesise...*

– learn the verb+prep combinations

Some words have developed partnerships with particular prepositions, especially for referring to activities or outcomes. The verb must be in the –ing form because of the preposition.

There is a tendency for writers to select the 'to+verb' form every time they are faced with this apparent 'choice'. Again, check the correct usage for specific terms if unsure.

*capable/incapable of – They are incapable ~~to form~~ (**of forming**) social networks in this environment.*

*succeed in – This may be more effective and actually succeed ~~to improve~~ (**in improving**) overall health.*

*suspected of – They were suspected ~~to have~~ (**of having**) an obstruction...*

CASE REPORT: LOSS OF INFINITIVE 'TO'

Sometimes the 'to' is missing from the infinitive form. This is most commonly seen after modal verbs and after an object when the main verb is hear, see, make or let.

A very common error is to retain the 'to' when these verbs feature.

The lack of sample size would ~~to~~ lead to a misinterpretation...

We would then make the nurse ~~to~~ check with other staff members.

Learn how to make the right choice

Here are some common dilemmas and their solutions:

To help with interpret/interpreting these scatter plots we used...

↓

The –ing form is required because the preceding word is a preposition (with).

This mistake is often seen when 'before', 'after' or 'since' begin a sentence:

Before ~~measure~~ *(**measuring**) the time it takes to...*

This requires change/changing the dose weekly so that...

↓

The verb 'to require' necessitates that the verbal following is in the –ing form.

The assay is designed to detect/detecting fusion transcripts...

↓

The endings of the infinitive form cannot change. It retains the dictionary form or plain form of the verb and is unaffected by tense or plurality. So 'detect' is required. Here is another example:

We hope ~~to evaluates~~ *(**to evaluate**) these measures at a later date.*

*The GP may then decide (**to**) refer the patient to a...*

↓

Remember to include the 'to' part

CASE REPORT: AN OBSTRUCTION BETWEEN THE MAIN VERB AND VERBAL

So far we have looked at sentences where the verbal follows the main verb with no other words in between.

*It **continued to produce** the best results.*

Some verbs require an actor (a pronoun or a noun) between the main verb and the verbal.

A verb that always causes problems is 'to allow'.

This will allow to calculate the p value. ✗

This will allow (us/them) to calculate the p value. ✓

Another option is to make the sentence passive: *This will allow.......to be calculated.*

The infinitive can immediately follow 'allow' if a form of the verb 'to be' has already helped to introduce the subject. Compare the following:

We allowed (the patients in groups 1 and 2) to apply this liberally.
actor required

Patients in groups 1 and 2 were allowed to apply this liberally.
actor already stated

Other verbs that require an 'actor' are advise, convince, enable, encourage, instruct, permit.

*We can then convince **the staff** to adopt these measures.*

*The researcher will then instruct **the patient** to apply the cream...*

Meet with the modals

Modals are auxiliary verbs that change the manner of a sentence and show the likelihood or ability of something. They are followed by a main verb and give extra information related to ability, possibility, necessity or willingness.

can/could   will/would   may/might/must   should/shall

The verb form that follows is always the infinitive but without the 'to'.

*This type of comparison group **can provide** normative data so...*

– remember two golden rules

A golden rule to follow when using modal verbs is that the verb immediately after the modal retains its base or dictionary form.

*The study **measures** the severity and type of...*

*The study **will measure** the severity and type of...*

So even when the subject is singular, the verb can take the same form as the plural when a modal verb is present.

*These strategies **improve** a person's motivation to eat a healthy diet.*   (plural)

*The strategy should **improve** a person's motivation to eat a healthy diet.*   (singular – same form with a modal)

*This would also ~~results~~ **(result)** in a higher number being screened.*

The second golden rule is (as already mentioned) the verb never changes, so the –ing form cannot be used after a modal.

*Free radicals can ~~causing~~ **(cause)** damage to people's bodies over time.*

– will/would

'Would' is incorrectly used by writers specifying what they plan to discuss in their work. Because of its role in conditional sentences, it sounds to the reader as though this was not actually possible.

We would choose this material for reconstruction.

The reader is waiting for the second part of the sentence...

*We would choose this material for reconstruction **but its suitability has yet to be confirmed.***

Instead, 'will' informs the reader what follows because the future tense is required.

*We **will** choose this material for reconstruction.*

*This **will** be covered in a later chapter.*

> The only time 'would' can be used in this context is to express hope or justification.
>
> *This study would be able to solve this problem.*
>
> *This would be valuable to patients who have little spare time.*

One issue that occurs with 'will' is the insertion of a past tense verb form.

*This will ~~facilitated~~ (**facilitate**) the drug development process.*

> The writer either wanted the sentence in the past tense and inserted 'will' by mistake, or used the past tense form of the verb instead of the standard form required for the future tense.

– can/could

Use **can** to describe something in the present or future that is likely or certain to happen or that you are able to do.

We can determine how long this will take by applying the curve...

Use **can** for seeking or granting permission.

They can leave the trial at any time by informing the facilitator stationed toward the back of the room.

Use **could** to describe something that is possible in the present or future, but may not happen for various reasons.

We could monitor each minor sensation but are restricted by time.

Use **could** to express alternatives or possible reasons.

They could also look at cases where the cause was an environmental one.

This could explain why the value is not significant.

'could' is the past tense of 'can' so is also used for past events.

They could fully rotate their shoulder before the second operation.

'Could' is often unnecessarily added in the present tense.

We ~~could~~ realise that the RQR value has changed in set...

– should

Use should when there is a reasonable expectation that something will happen.

They should be able to detect a change within a few days.

Use should for making recommendations about your own study or future studies.

These therapies should be included especially for post-surgery patients.

– may

Use may to report something cautiously and where doubt is involved.

It may even involve the whole gastro-intestinal tract...

CASE REPORT: QUESTIONNAIRES

Questions contain auxiliary verbs ('be', 'do', 'have') or/and modals. Sometimes these verbs are missed out in error.

How many children you have? (missing 'do')

They meet the emotional and relational needs?
(missing 'Can')

In questions the modal verb comes before the subject.

Can they improve on their postnatal care?

In a statement the subject comes first.

They can improve on their postnatal care.

In questions 'would' is used for offers and requests.

Would you like more information?

In questions 'can' is used to ask permission or make a suggestion while 'could' is a more polite form.

Could I use this data for my research?

In questions 'may' is used to ask for permission formally.

May I offer my opinion?

Modals can be changed to negatives by adding 'not'. This is placed between the modal and the main verb. In informal writing negatives can be shortened with an apostrophe, but this is not recommended for academic writing.

could not (couldn't)   will not (won't)   should not (shouldn't)

These parameters ~~won't~~ *(**will not**) be suitable for those with compromised vision.*

Appreciate the abstract nature of phrasal verbs

Phrasal verbs are multi-part verbs made up of a verb and a preposition or particle. They are different to other phrases that contain prepositions in that the meaning is not obvious if the parts of the phrasal verb are considered separately.

*The reviews **point out** the weakness of this particular study.*

These verbs end in directional words such as 'on', 'down', 'out' and 'back' but they are being used in an abstract way, so judging them can be difficult. Many phrasal verbs are considered colloquial or examples of informal language, so single-word verbs are preferable (e.g. start off – begin); but some have an important part to play in medical writing and are certainly useful as descriptive terms once their meaning has been acquired and use mastered.

act on/upon	add on	back down
break away	break down	break through
break up	bring down about	bring up
build up	cancel out	come across
come back	come up with	cough up
cover up	cut off	cut out
depend on	drop off	drop out
ease off	fall back on	get around
help out	look into	look after
pass by	pass on	pass out
phase out	rule out	scale down
set up	shut down	team up
tell apart	tune in to	turn on/off
turn up/down	type in	use up

– position of the small part of the phrase

The position of the second word in some of these verbs is fixed, coming directly after the verb and before the object.

*Six participants **dropped out** of the study at the second stage.*

In other verbs the position is flexible.

*We can therefore **rule** this **out** as a possible cause.*

*We can **rule out** the possibility of...*

– types of error: confusion with single-word verbs

Some writers confuse two-word verbs with single-word verbs that are similar in meaning. Other writers overlook the single-word verb, which, if available, should always be chosen over a phrasal. (see also Complaint L)

*To ensure this does not ~~spread out~~ **(spread)**, measures must be taken not only on the ward but...*

*It would be useful to ~~find out~~ **(discover)** why group B did not.*

*Unfortunately this further ~~held up~~ **(delayed)** the procedure.*

*Twelve out of 80 were ~~left out~~ **(omitted)** from the analysis.*

*They ~~tried out~~ **(tested)** the procedure to ensure that...*

– wrong particle

*Currently, government policies ~~focus in~~ **(focus on)** helping those who want to quit.*

*Much will ~~depend with~~ **(depend on)** the location of the...*

*This was ~~phased away~~ **(phased out)** in the 1980s.*

– confusion between particles

Some phrasal verbs contain the same verb but have a different particle and therefore a different meaning.

*Further trials will be ~~carried on~~ **(carried out)** with this in mind.* (see also a–z)

*The nurses ~~came up with~~ **(came up against)** a number of senior administrators who were not prepared to listen.*

*This group was asked to ~~cut off~~ (**cut out**) dairy for a week.*

*We suggest that they provide information about the participants who ~~dropped off~~ (**dropped out**).*

INTERVENTION   **questionnaires and forms**

Questionnaires and forms can be filled out or filled in but not just filled.

These questionnaires were filled by the parents.   ✗

– result in/from

result in – to lead to   result from – to be caused by

*These hormonal changes **resulted in** lower concentrations…*

*There are 58 recognised structures relating to swelling, **resulting from** a specific reaction of antibodies…*

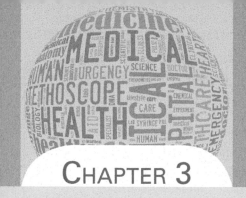

CHAPTER 3

Complaint C: Adjectives and adverbs

Signs:
→ Inability to choose between adjectives and adverbs
→ Problems with choosing a suitable description
→ Failing to realise which quantifiers take singular and plural nouns and verbs

Treatment

Adjectives only ever modify nouns and pronouns. Adverbs are more flexible and can provide information about verbs, adjectives and other adverbs. The most common decision facing a writer here is whether to use the adjective or the related adverb ending in –ly (note not all adverbs end in –ly).

This has been temporary/temporarily used to relieve pain.

The word is modifying a verb (use) and so an adverb will be required – temporarily.

ASSESSMENT		adjectives for shapes
circular	cylindrical	add –ly to form the adverb
linear	orthogonal	add –ity for the noun form
rectangular	triangular	
pyramidal	conical	

> **ASSESSMENT**   **patient description vs. symptoms**
>
> Adjectives 'describe' and nouns 'name'.
> *The gum is* **sensitive**   (description) – adjective
> *There is* **sensitivity** *in the gum*
> (name of the state or condition) – noun
>
> So the adjective will be required here.
> *The experimental group is gluten* ~~sensitivity~~ (**sensitive**).
>
> *The patient felt* **restless** *all of the time*   – adjective
> **Restlessness** *is also experienced*   – noun

Learn the endings
Is it -ory or -ary?

ambulatory ~~ambulatary~~   inspiratory
auditory   mammary ~~mammory~~
axillary ~~axillory~~   olfactory
biliary   pituitary
capillary   pulmonary ~~pulmonory~~
ciliary   refractory
circulatory ~~circulatary~~   respiratory ~~respiratary~~
coronary   salivary
dietary   sensory
excretory ~~excretary~~   urinary
expiratory ~~expiratary~~   ventilatory ~~ventilatary~~
inflammatory

So adjectives can often be determined by their endings or suffixes. However, it would be wrong to assume that all terms with these endings are adjectives.

> *Also/*
> *hereditary   primary   secondary*
> *stationary   temporary   tertiary*

memory – noun   ovary – noun   suppository – noun

Is it -al or -ar?

abdominal	glandular
arterial	jugular
articular	molecular
artificial	muscular
atrial	musculoskeletal
aural (relating to the ear)	neurological
bacterial	nodal
cardial (see a–z)	occular
cardiovascular	oral (relating to the mouth)
cellular	peritoneal
cerebral	pleural
clinical	renal
congenital	surgical
cranial	tracheal
dentinal	vascular
facial	ventricular
fungal	venular
gastrointestinal	

Adjectives of general location tend to end in –al.

central	internal	medial	regional
distal	lateral	peripheral	terminal
external	local	proximal	

How about –ic?

acoustic	gastric	peptic
aerobic	genetic	prosthetic
aortic	hepatic	psychiatric
cardiogenic	lactic	rheumatic
chronic	metabolic	systolic
cystic	metastatic	thoracic
diuretic	orthopaedic	traumatic
ectopic	pelvic	trophic

Also/	automatic	diagnostic	episodic
	extrinsic	intrinsic	symptomatic

Noun/adjective confusion is widespread in English. Many cases involve the endings –nce (for nouns) and –nt (for adjectives). Compare the following:

NOUN(-nce)	ADJECTIVE(-nt)		
absence	absent (see a–z)	inconvenience	inconvenient
absorbance	absorbant	persistence	persistent
adherence	adherent	presence	present
		prevalence (see a–z)	prevalent
adolescence	adolescent	prominence	prominent
compliance	compliant	resistance	resistant
confidence	confident	resonance	resonant
difference	different	significance	significant
fluorescence	flourescent	tolerance (see a–z)	tolerant
importance	important	variance	variant
incidence	incident	virulence	virulent

But the following have a different noun form:

consistency	consistent
deficiency	deficient (see a–z)
pregnancy	pregnant

Words ending in –nt may not always be adjectives. Two of the adjectives in the list above can also be nouns.

*The first **incident** had occurred six weeks earlier.*

*But this related to an **adolescent** who had a history of mental impairment.*

Put the adverb in its place

Adverbs are most effective when appearing before the modified word, and they have to be placed there when that word is an adjective.

*This was **significantly changed** with the addition of Raftiline.*

But adverbs that describe how something is done, adverbs of time and adverbial phrases can be found after the modified word and at the end of a sentence.

*The pH in the upper small intestine **decreases slowly** after meal intake (33).*

*The clinic would then forward these **at a later date**.*

When forms of 'to be' are involved, the adverb comes after the verb.

*The femoral approach **is frequently** used during trauma resuscitation.*

As a rule, adverbs should be placed as close to the word being modified as possible to avoid confusion and ambiguity.

*We **frequently use** this source to ensure that our...*

Know how to compare

Adjectives and adverbs can be used to compare things and there are three degrees of comparison.

attribute degree –	high	likely(+)	likely(–)	good
comparative degree –	higher	more likely	less likely	better
superlative degree –	highest	most likely*	least likely	best

The comparative degree compares two things and the superlative degree compares at least three. Most adjectives and adverbs take on the forms above as they move through the comparative stages. Notice however that 'good' has an irregular construction and different words are used to create the comparison.

*This tendon has a **high** pain threshold.*

*This tendon has a **higher** pain threshold than the distal end of the fibula.*

*This tendon has the **highest** pain threshold of all those tested.*

> This was the ~~lower~~ (**lowest**) SCFA producer of all the cereals tested.

---

* Not 'most possible'.

Some adjectives cannot form these different degrees of comparison by changing their endings, so they use more/less and most/least instead. A common error is failing to recognize the ones that can.

*The bacterium also showed the ~~most close~~ (**closest**) association with low colon cancer risk.*

Note also how 'than' is used to complete the comparative form. Adjectives in the first degree do not technically compare so cannot be used with 'than'.

The results of this treatment are disappointing ~~than~~ the standard procedure of root planning…

So if there is not a comparing word in the sentence 'than' should not be used. 'Compared with' can be used to form a comparison instead.

*The results of this treatment are disappointing **compared with** the standard procedure of root planing, which achieved…*

When there is an apparent choice between the two terms, opt for 'than' if the adjective is in the comparative degree and the two things are being evaluated directly.

*Efficiency in the transfected cells was also much greater ~~compared with~~ (**than**) in the control cells.*

INTERVENTION   **comparatively little**

Use small for the actual size of something not little.
*These brown spots are relatively ~~little~~ (**small**).*
Little in size does not have satisfactory comparatives.
Little in amount follows the order little, less, least.

It is important to consider whether the reader will be able to identify what is being compared. It might seem obvious to the writer but has the comparison actually been formed?

Men with a higher myricetin intake have a lower risk of prostate cancer.

> Higher than who?   How high?

Get past the past participle

Present and past participles can function as adjectives. Past participles that end in –ed (many of them do) are often unwittingly written without the 'd' when paired with nouns.

*We will also demonstrate three types of ~~balance~~ (**balanced**) diets that are currently...*

*There were a number of issues with the ~~estimate~~ (**estimated**) recovery times.*

Are your adjectives excessive?

Adjectives and adverbs should be used thoughtfully and only for description or emphasis. Do not use robust adjectives to persuade the reader of something or overemphasize a situation. Strong adjectives usually sound unprofessional, inappropriate and give the impression that the writer is trying too hard to convince the reader. Use more modest adjectives and phrases that have clear and direct meanings and that the reader will be more familiar with and will more likely accept.

*~~An incredible~~ (**A key**) observation is that once a patient has...*

*It also led to a ~~magnificent~~ (**marked**) decrease in lost data.*

*There is a ~~massive~~ (**large**) amount of research on this topic...*

This is ~~absolutely~~ crucial to the success of the scheme.

Compare specific terms
– small/few/little

'little' can precede uncountable nouns when referring to amount. For physical size use 'small' instead (see final example).

Little evidence *was found to support this view.*

'few' can precede plural nouns when referring to number.

Few patients *were aware of the potential dangers involved.*

'small' cannot go directly before the noun when referring to amount or number.

~~Small evidence~~ has been collected already.

Only when it is relating to the actual size of something can it go next to the noun.

Small *polyps may still not be detected by this test.*

– less/fewer

less – not as much
fewer – not as many

Use fewer with countable nouns.

*...where there are ~~less~~ (**fewer**) nephrons than normal.*

So side effects will require fewer not less.

*Naturally, the aim was for the drug to produce **fewer** of these side effects.*

Use less with uncountable nouns.

*They documented much **less** bleeding after the procedure.*

Recognise other errors

First, the normally-hearing individuals were asked to...   ✗

> Be careful which terms you use as modifiers. Here 'individuals with normal hearing' is appropriate.

Their study involved Swedish young men with...   ✗

> When using consecutive adjectives, the person's age must come before their nationality or ethnicity.
>
> *Their study involved young Swedish men with...*

*The study highlighted the importance of a less ~~stress~~ (**stressful**) lifestyle and...*

*From the data provided, it is ~~clearly~~ (**clear**) that patients with a high residual volume are at risk.*

*They also found it to be ~~inverse~~ (**inversely**) correlated with the risk of cardiovascular disease.*

*We looked at the strategies of various NHS ~~organisation~~ (**organisations**)...*

> 'various' modifies a plural noun not a singular countable.

*This medication performed twice as fast ~~than~~ (**as**) the previous one.*

> This sentence uses an adjective in the first degree (fast) so 'than' cannot be used. However, a comparative construction is possible by using the following form:
>
> *as + adjective + as*

*We followed the DSM –IV criteria (which is the ~~last~~ (**latest**) version)...*

> Last implies end or final version so latest would be a better choice here.

Learn which quantifiers are singular/plural

Quantifiers come before the noun and modify it. They are usually used instead of articles.

~~The~~ each method has its merits as a potential solution.

Others like little, most, and few can have articles before them. Take note of the difference in meaning with and without an article.

*There was **little** loss of accuracy here.*

(almost none – positive outcome)

*There was **a little** loss of accuracy here.*

(some – negative outcome)

***Few studies** have looked at this topic.*

(not many studies – negative)

***A few studies** have looked at this topic.* (some – positive)

When these words are the subject of the sentence it is always difficult to know whether to use a singular or plural verb. Some take singular, some plural and others both. It is also difficult to know whether they take countable or uncountable nouns. Here is a list of quantifiers along with some other words that imply quantity and the nouns and verbs they take.

all – sing or plural verb; plural or uncountable noun, e.g.

> *All training **was** carried out during the...*
>
> *All values **were** normalised to ensure...*
>
> *All **patients** had taken this drug for three weeks...*
>
> *All of the **evidence** indicates that environmental factors...*

another – singular verb; singular countable noun

any – singular or plural verb; singular, plural or uncountable noun

both – plural verb; plural noun

each – singular verb; singular countable noun

either – singular verb; singular countable noun

enough – plural verb; plural or uncountable noun

few – plural verb; plural noun

little – singular verb; uncountable noun

many – plural verb; plural noun

more – singular or plural verb; plural or uncountable noun

most – sing or plural verb; plural or uncountable noun

much – singular verb; uncountable noun

neither – singular verb; singular countable noun

other – singular or plural verb; plural or uncountable noun

several – plural verb; plural noun

some – singular or plural verb; plural or uncountable noun

these – plural verb; plural noun

those – plural verb; plural noun

Recognise the meaning of the 'of' phrase

The phrase 'of the' can be used between a quantifier and a noun. By doing this the noun can take on a definite meaning.

In **most of the** cases bone overgrowth was observed in that area. (definite: The specific cases being studied)

In **most cases** bone overgrowth is observed in that area. (indefinite: Cases in general)

All of the nurses must fill out these forms when...

(definite: A specific group)

All nurses must fill out these forms when...

(indefinite: Nurses in general)

Note the errors

For each ~~reactions~~ (**reaction**) 45 cycles were performed.

> 'each' is always singular so will have a singular noun and a singular form of the verb to be.

Each task ~~were~~ (**was**) performed at a controlled cadence of 0.4 Hz using a metronome.

This was demonstrated to be effective in both acute and community ~~setting~~ (**settings**).

> 'both' is always linked with a plural noun.

Much of the evidence ~~were~~ (**was**) ignored because of weak administration within the...

> Here an uncountable noun has been used with 'much'. This is fine, but the verb must then be singular.

*One of the ~~hypothesis~~ (**hypotheses**) related to...*

*In the next chapter we demonstrate that these are ~~genetic~~ (**genetically**) determined.*

*They had ~~fewer~~ (**less**) data than Morgan and thus the reliability of the outcome was questioned...*

> Data is an unusual noun in that it can be considered either singular or plural and also has an uncountable meaning. Less and little are used with data as well as quantity phrases such as 'piece of' and 'amount of'.

*Numerous ~~study~~ (**studies**) have assessed whether a hayfever sufferer should...*

Not only was it ~~much~~ successful in simulating the in vivo plasma profile, but it was also ~~very~~ important for assessing...

*We then assessed the ~~health~~ (**healthy**) participants...*

*Indeed, an increase approximately 3-fold greater ~~then~~ (**than**) the control cells was observed...*

*A score of 10 represented the ~~worse~~ (**worst**) possible discomfort.*

> As with good/better/best, the example above shows another set of irregular comparatives being used. Bad is the initial attribute, worse is the comparative term and worst is the superlative.

> ## CASE REPORT: DON'T BE ALL NEGATIVE
>
> Sometimes 'all' begins a sentence that is negative in nature.
> A better construction is to begin with 'no/none'.
>
> *All the subjects do not exercise regularly.* ✗
> *None of the subjects exercise regularly.* ✓
>
> Another issue is when the writer actually means 'only some'. For this, 'not all' can be used.
>
> *All of the subjects do not have a family history of this.* ✗
> *Not all of the subjects have a family history of this.* ✓
>
> For negation use 'any' not 'all' to mean none. In the sentence below 'all' would imply that it still worked on some of the subjects.
>
> *This did not work for ~~all~~ (**any**) of the subjects.*

– another/other

For countable nouns use the terms in the following way:

another – singular (one other; a further)

other – plural (some other; further)

*~~Other~~ (**Another**) study **has** focused on the shortcomings of the traditional treatment plan...*

*~~Another~~ (**Other**) studies **have** focused on the shortcomings of the traditional treatment plan...*

– as well /also

'as well' normally goes at the end of a sentence.

*This gene could play an important part **as well**.*

It can only go at the beginning in the form 'As well as...'

*As **well** as providing individual support, it **also** benefitted the other residents.*

'as well' is always two words.   ~~aswell~~

'Also' can appear at the beginning of a clause as a conjunctive adverb,

*...~~as well~~, **(also,)** there was very little funding available.*

or be used as an adverb modifying verbs and adjectives.

*This could ~~as well~~ **(also)** affect the original parameters.*

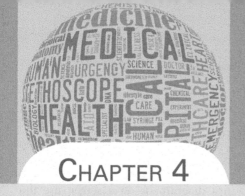

CHAPTER 4

Complaint D: Prepositions

Signs:
→ Finding it difficult to choose among the prepositions

Treatment

There are few general rules relating to preposition choice and it can be difficult to work out which preposition should be used in a given situation or with a certain term. That said, there are a few situations where the logic is apparent (see also Complaint G).

Physically, 'in' is used for indicating that something is contained within something else.

*These were then placed **in** containers until needed.*

While 'on' is used for something on a surface or just above.

*The files were placed **on the table** for the students to inspect.*

Also, use 'in' for months and years.

*This occurred **in** June.   This occurred **in** June 2014.*
*This occurred **in** 2009.*

And use 'on' for specific dates and days of the week.

*This occurred **on** June 15th 2014*

*This occurred (~~in~~) **on** Tuesday.*

When referring to position in a diagram or on a screen use the following:

at *the top*   **in** *the middle*   **at** *the bottom*

---

in (a liquid)   **at** (a temperature)   **for** (a time)

*The membrane was incubated **in** 3% skimmed milk*
***at** 37°C **for** 1h.*

ASSESSMENT   **preps for anatomy**

around/in the mouth	**in** the ears
on/in/up the nose	**on** the skin
on/between the toes	**on/between** the fingers
around/in the eyes	**in** the stomach
on the knee	**on/under** the arms
in the hair	**on** the scalp
on the hands	**on** the feet

– among/between

'Between' is generally used to refer to two things.

This included an analysis of the relationship between smoking and obesity.

'Among' is used for more than two.

We also measured its popularity among the patients with ME.

CASE REPORT: HOSPITAL

The noun hospital is quite versatile in the prepositions it can take. That said, specific situations will require specific prepositions and a choice is not generally available.

*When a patient is **in** hospital it is important for them to feel...*

Here a definite article is not required. The 'in hospital' is considered a fixed phrase.

*The patient was taken **to** hospital/to the hospital.*

The definite article is optional here. Like school and other familiar institutions the definite article can be dropped from the noun.

*The trial was carried out **at** Fairfield Hospital over the course of two weeks.*

Use 'at' when referring to the hospital as the location for something.

Learn the prepositional phrases

Given their rather abstract nature and the numerous definitions they attract, the most effective way to learn prepositions is to become familiar with the words and phrases they form relationships with. Those terms most commonly found in medical papers and most often misused are listed here. The following boxes list the terms by preposition needed and then the examples are listed by alphabetical order of the term they form a relationship with.

Arranged by preposition

BY
accompanied by
caused by
characterised by
complicated by
exacerbated by
hindered by
induced by
precipitated by
relieved by
stimulated by
transmitted by
verified by

WITH
In accordance with
associated with
in combination with
combined with
compatible with
in conjunction with
contact with
interfere with

FROM
arising from
benefit from
derive from
die from
relief from

OF
avoidance of
of benefit
cause of
composed of
consist of
degree of
diagnostic of
history of
incidence of
independent of
indicative of
likelihood of
limitation of
perception of
at risk of
suggestive of
symptomatic of

FOR
accounts for
adjusted for
controlling for
eligible for
examine for
need for
reason for
responsible for
screened for
tested…for

TO
adhere to
admitted to
allocated to
alternative to
assigned to
attributed to
aversion to
confined to
contribute to
exposure to
to some extent
obstacle to
point to
predisposed to
prior to
prone to
resistant to
responsive to
sensitive to
subject to
susceptible to
vulnerable to

ON
on average
depend on
impact on
on occasion
rely on

IN
in the absence of
in adulthood
in the long term
in origin

—in the absence of

~~With~~ (**In**) the absence of symptoms, this should be managed carefully...

> ~~In the absent of...~~

—accompanied by

This is usually accompanied ~~with~~ (**by**) nausea and vomiting.

—in accordance with

This is in accordance ~~to~~ (**with**) our previous findings.

—accounts for

It accounts ~~to~~ (**for**) 60% of premature deaths worldwide.

—adhere to

Patients were also asked to adhere ~~with~~ (**to**) a low-sodium diet.

—adjusted for

The models that were adjusted ~~to~~ (**for**) covariates appear in Table 8 and Table 9.

> statistical adjustment of data uses 'adjusted for'

—admitted to

In this case they would be admitted ~~in~~ (**to**) an ITU.

—in adulthood/childhood

~~At~~ (**In**) adulthood the risk decreases considerably...

—allocated to

In total, twenty subjects were allocated ~~in~~ (**to**) the control group.

> When placing into groups use 'allocated to';
> when referring to time use 'allocated for'

—alternative to

A possible alternative ~~with~~ (**to**) bone repair could be this subcutaneous adipose tissue.

—under anaesthesia

*The bone defects were created by the extraction previously described in six non-human primates ~~in~~ (**under**) general anaesthesia.*

—arising from

*They assessed injuries of the ear arising ~~to~~ (**from**) fractures of the skull.*

—assigned to

*Participants who meet the inclusion criteria will be randomly assigned ~~with~~ (**to**) either the experimental group or the control group.*

—associated with

*The former appears to be associated ~~to~~ (**with**) a reduced incidence of IBS.*

—attributed to

*This is attributed ~~in~~ (**to**) their consumption of spicy food.*

on average (see also a–z)

*~~In~~ (**On**) average, the limb volume increases by around 25%.*

—aversion to

*This is a particularly useful scheme for those with an aversion ~~about~~ (**to**) exercise.*

—avoidance of

*This includes avoidance ~~to~~ (**of**) excess noise and high frequencies if possible.*

—benefit from (see also a–z)

*The study suggests that they might also benefit ~~for~~ (**from**) alternative treatment methods.*

—of benefit

*Certain anti-inflammatory agents have been shown to be ~~in~~ (**of**) benefit.*

—cause of (see also a–z)

*They researched whether lipid peroxidation was a cause ~~to~~ (**of**) lower limb swelling.*

> BUT/ The speed at which the rash spread is certainly a **cause for** concern.

—caused by

*The health issues presented were likely to be caused from (**by**) age-related changes.*

—characterised by

*This is a multisystem disorder characterised with (**by**) inflammation...*

—in combination with

*Issues with microcirculation in combination of (**with**) atherosclerosis lead to...*

—combined with

*Combined to (**with**) other drugs this has the potential to offer an attractive short term solution.*

—compatible with

*The examination and biopsies revealed inflammation in this area that was compatible to (**with**) Crohn's disease.*

—complicated by

*As before, the situation is often complicated from (**by**) secondary infection.*

—composed of

*The system is composed by (**of**) three genes located on human chromosome 9.*

> composed by = created by

—confined to

*This condition is usually confined by (**to**) the kidneys and is an important factor in...*

—in conjunction with

*Gas retention in conjunction to (**with**) stress may produce visible abdominal distension.*

—consist of

*The assays consist ~~with~~ (**of**) a pair of unlabelled sequence-specific primers that...*

—constitute

Although these cases are rare, they still constitute ~~of~~ an important group...

—contact with

*Transmission occurs by contact ~~to~~ (**with**) an infested individual or material such as bedding.*

—contribute to

*These mechanisms have also been shown to contribute ~~in~~ (**to**) hyperemia.*

—controlling for

*They studied the effects of coping on psychological outcome when controlling ~~of~~ (**for**) background variables.*

> 'Controlling for' relates to statistically checking or regulating variables.

—degree of

*The degree ~~in~~ (**of**) pulmonary stenosis was mild in both cases.*

—depend on

*The effects depend ~~with~~ (**on**) their concentration in the diet and the amount consumed.*

—derive from

*These deposits may be derived ~~of~~ (**from**) the circulation in the kidney.*

—diagnostic of (see also a–z)

*However, a score of ≥5 was diagnostic ~~for~~ (**of**) Stickler syndrome.*

—die from

*They found that the majority died ~~with~~ (**from**) complications arising from hypertension, particularly heart disease and...*

—eligible for (see also a–z)

Patients were eligible ~~in~~ inclusion if they were 50 years of age or above and...

—exacerbated by

In almost all cases the pain is exacerbated ~~with~~ (by) sudden movement such as coughing and sneezing.

—examine for

To examine ~~in~~ (for) rectal disease it may be necessary to carry out a sigmoidoscopy.

—exposure to

Exposure ~~with~~ (to) contaminated food must also be considered.

—to some/a lesser/greater extent

The prognosis has improved ~~in~~ (to) some extent...

—hindered by

Recovery could also be hindered ~~with~~ (by) the lack of a support network.

—history of

We also checked for a history ~~with~~ (of) psychiatric illness.

—impact on

Ethnic origin may impact ~~to~~ (on) gut function and gut microbiota colonisation...

—incidence of

They reported a low incidence ~~from~~ (of) postoperative pneumonia.

—independent of

...might be responsible for the rise in obesity, independent ~~from~~ (of) level of physical activity.

—indicative of

This is indicative ~~for~~ (of) partial or complete catheter blockage.

—induced by

This alteration can be induced ~~with~~ (by) a traumatic event...

—interfere with

These elements are unlikely to interfere ~~on~~ (with) bowel cleansing.

—likelihood of

*The risk factors that increase the likelihood ~~for~~ (**of**) pneumonia are listed in Table 5.*

—limitation of

*The main limitation ~~for~~ (**of**) this study is the lack of a control group.*

—In the long/short term

*~~On~~ (**In**) the long term, the effects on bone health will be...*

—need for

*These results highlight the need ~~of~~ (**for**) studies to test whether pyloric drainage can effectively prevent reflux symptoms.*

> 'need of' is used with 'in' and as a plural.
>
> *The clinic is **in need of** a modern IT system.*
>
> *We must address the **needs of** these marginal groups.*

—an obstacle to

*It can be considered an obstacle ~~of~~ (**to**) applying this approach in casework.*

—on... occasion

*We chose to carry this out ~~in~~ (**on**) two separate occasions to confirm the initial findings.*

—in origin

*These tumours are monoclonal ~~on~~ (**in**) origin but there is little evidence to suggest that...*

—perception of

*Next we assess their perception ~~to~~ (**of**) pain using the following scale:*

—point to

*These all point ~~at~~ (**to**) a distinct lack of iron in their diet and limited...*

> 'point to' means to indicate or suggest

—precipitated by

*This can be precipitated ~~from~~ (**by**) events such as oral contraceptive therapy and the menopause.*

> 'precipitated by' means brought about by

—predisposed to (see also a–z)

*Studies have shown that women are predisposed ~~of~~ (**to**) autoimmune rheumatic diseases.*

> 'predisposed to' means 'susceptible to' or to have a tendency towards

—prior to

*Even being overweight or obese prior (**to**) pregnancy is linked to increased risk of...*

—prone to

*These impairments make older people prone ~~for~~ (**to**) health problems that require unique health care.*

—reason for

*One reason ~~of~~ (**for**) this is the difficulty in measuring fermentation in vivo.*

—relief from (see also a–z)

*It is effective in providing relief ~~of~~ (**from**) bloating.*

—relieved by

*The pain can be relieved ~~from~~ (**by**) antiinflammatory drugs and injection with...*

—rely on

*This mechanism may rely ~~in~~ (**on**) the presence of other contributing factors such as damage to specific cells...*

—resistant to

*Most of the compounds that are resistant ~~of~~ (**to**) acid hydrolysis in the stomach pass to the colon.*

—responsible for

*The pacemaker is responsible ~~in~~ (**for**) maintaining ventricular contractions...*

Also: responsible to (a person or group of people)

—responsive to

*Aggressive lymphomas are more responsive ~~with~~ (**to**) chemotherapy but have...*

—at risk of/for

*Patients would also be ~~in~~ (**at**) risk of secondary infection.*

—screened for

*The residents in each nursing home were screened ~~of~~ (**for**) suitability based on the selection criteria.*

—sensitive to

*When grown in oxygen they were more sensitive ~~for~~ (**to**) oxidative stress...*

—stimulated by (see also a–z *simulate*)

*They studied whether the growth of this intestinal bacterium is stimulated ~~from~~ (**by**) dietary flavonoids in vivo.*

—subject to

*The contents were then subjected ~~for~~ (**to**) extreme temperatures before...*

'subject to' means to undergo or experience something

—suggestive of

*The nature of this tenderness was strongly suggestive ~~for~~ (**of**) pyelonephritis.*

—susceptible to

*The theory is that outer hair cells are more susceptible ~~for~~ (**to**) damage than inner hair cells.*

—symptomatic of

As epilepsy is possibly symptomatic ~~to~~ (of) an underlying brain disorder...

—tested for (see also a–z *result*)

The patient had tested positive ~~to~~ (for) hepatitis C.

—transmitted by

This rare infectious disease is mostly transmitted ~~from~~ (by) the ingestion of shellfish.

—verified by

This will be developed and verified ~~with~~ (by) the research team and relevant experts.

—vulnerable to

It can explain why these individuals might be vulnerable ~~from~~ (to) developing a food addiction.

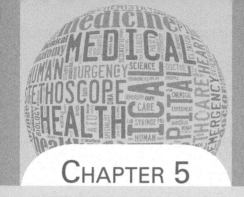

CHAPTER 5

Complaint E: Clauses

Signs:
→ Failing to appreciate dependent clauses
→ Using the wrong connecting words
→ Creating sentences with the wrong construction

Treatment

Every sentence has a main clause that contains a subject and a verb. Main clauses are also known as independent clauses because they can stand on their own without needing any additional information. They represent a complete idea or thought.

The patients were followed for five years.

A dependent clause depends on the independent (main) clause for its meaning so it cannot be used on its own. It is only part of a sentence and not a complete thought.

Which could prove difficult in the long run.

This clause cannot stand on its own as it is an incomplete thought.

Recognise the clause categories

There are two kinds of dependent clause, conditional and relative.

– conditional clauses

Conditional clauses talk about things that will, could or might happen now or in the future. They can also talk about things that could have happened in the past. They usually begin with 'if' or 'unless'.

If we turn our attention to the inheritance we can immediately see discrepancies related to phenotype 3.

This is the most effective test to use **unless there is contraindication...**

– relative clauses

Relative clauses start with relative pronouns such as *that, which, whichever, who, whoever* and *whose*.

We assessed the starch **that was recovered from the effluent.**

There are two types of relative clause.

- A restrictive or essential relative clause influences the meaning of the sentence and cannot be left out.

  She was the carer **who had looked after both women.**

- A nonrestrictive or nonessential relative clause just gives extra information to the reader and if it is left out the sentence will still make sense.

  We were unable to detect an increase in COX-2 protein level, **which is consistent with previous studies.**

A comma always separates a nonrestrictive relative clause from the main clause. If the relative clause is in the middle of the sentence, then commas are used on either side.

We turned on the device, **which took about ten seconds***, and began the test.*

CASE REPORT: ALTHOUGH

One of the most common mistakes occurs with the conjunction 'although'.

Many writers put a comma after 'although' when it is part of a dependent clause at the start of a sentence.

Although, they are known to have low-transfection efficiency, they have been proven to generate reliable results.

If a comma is used directly after 'although' it is difficult for the reader to follow the meaning of the sentence. A comma indicates a pause and there should not be one here.

'although' can be used in a non-essential relative clause between commas like this,

*The literature on this topic, **although** extensive, is widely scattered.*

Do not use 'but' to link to the main clause when beginning with 'although' (or 'even though').

Although the sample was large, ~~but~~ the results proved inconclusive.

Select the correct conjunctions

There are two types of conjunction used with clauses, coordinating and subordinating.

Coordinating conjunctions join independent clauses to form a single sentence.

and, but, for, nor, or, so, yet

HO-1 has generally been considered as having antioxidant activity, but there is evidence it may be pro-oxidant.

> Subordinating conjunctions are used to begin dependent clauses.
>
> after, although, as, because, even if, even though, if, since, unless, whereas...
>
> *It would not be appropriate in this study, unless the patients had a mild form...*

Understand the conditions

As stated earlier, dependent clauses that begin with 'if' or 'unless' are known as conditional clauses. This is because a certain condition must be met before the action in the independent or main clause can occur. These conditions can be probable, possible in theory or even impossible.

> Conditional sentences may involve a prediction or opinion, or a clear intention to do something depending on a particular situation or action.

Probable – *If they enrol in the program, they will receive treatment tailored to their individual requirement.*

Possible – *If they enrolled in the program, they would receive treatment tailored to their individual requirement.*

Impossible (past) – *If they had enrolled in the program, they would have received treatment tailored to their individual requirement.*

The main error with 'probable' conditionals is using 'will' in the if-clause instead of the main clause.

If they ~~will~~ go a prolonged period without drinking, they will suffer similar problems...

Master other constructions
– comparative construction

A rather curiously formed but nevertheless frequently applied construction is this comparative one:

The longer the interval, the lower the overall density.

Both parts begin with 'the' and the verb 'to be' is often omitted. These are the four most common misconstructions:

The higher is the rating, the better quality of life is in that dimension.   ✗

The higher the rating is, the better is the quality of life in that dimension.   ✗

The higher the rating, better the quality of life in that dimension.   ✗

The higher rating, the better quality of life in that dimension.   ✗

The higher the rating, the better the quality of life in that dimension.   ✓

CASE REPORT: HOW LONG HAVE YOU HAD 'THAT' PROBLEM?

It is always difficult to know when to leave out 'that' and when to retain it.

When the 'that' is attached to the object of a noun clause it can be omitted.

The participants entered the rooms ~~that~~ they had been assigned to.

Read the sentence with and without 'that'. This should determine whether it can be omitted or not.

When 'that' is acting as the subject in an adjective clause (meaning it is part of a phrase modifying the noun) then it cannot be omitted.

*The next step is to reduce the lateral neurons **(that)** were previously excited.*

– only...

There are two constructions involving 'only' that can pose problems. The first one is a conditional that begins 'only if'.

When 'only if' begins a sentence the subject and verb are inverted (the same applies to 'only then' at the end of a sentence).

Only if they hear a noise they will press the button.   ✗

*Only if they hear a noise **will they** press the button.* ✓

The second is when a sentence begins with 'not only'. Again, note the differences between the two errors and the correct form. The first part is inverted but the second part is not.

Not only ~~they must~~ have knowledge of the different strategies, but ~~also they must~~ have enough influence to impose a scheme.

Not only ~~they must~~ have knowledge of the different strategies, ~~they also must~~ have enough influence to impose a scheme.

*Not only **must they** have knowledge of the different strategies, but **they must also** have enough influence to impose a scheme.*

Another construction is 'not only….but also'.

*We need to determine **not only** the fermentation of the different sources **but also** their digestibility before fermentation.*

Recognise the errors

Based on the results of these depletion experiments. We conclude that Bach1 inhibition has no protective role in the process. ↑

Here we have a dependent clause standing on its own. It is not a complete sentence, only an introductory phrase, so a comma is required not a period.

Because the research is only interested in the experiences of the patients, ~~so~~ the staff members will not be interviewed. ↑

A coordinating conjunction is not necessary when linking a dependent clause with an independent one.

Whereas histomorphological analysis took place twelve months after surgery; x-ray analyses were carried out at 1, 3 and 6 months.

> Do not use a semi colon to separate a dependent clause from an independent one. Use a comma instead.

The discomfort can be great and then the patient will normally be advised to change to a higher dose.

> The two independent clauses do not coordinate well. The first clause should be changed to a dependent one to act subordinately to the second part.
>
> *When the discomfort is great, the patient will normally be advised to change to a higher dose.*

Paediatrics is a branch of medicine, which focuses on infants, children and adolescents.

> Here a clause has been broken up too early with a comma and 'which'. This implies a non-essential clause when in fact the main clause should just continue with 'that' and no comma.
>
> *Paediatrics is a branch of medicine that focuses on infants, children and adolescents.*

Since the test was based on two levels, ~~but~~ only the second region criteria needed to be satisfied.

> Again, no need for the linking word here.

Abrasion can be differentiated from attrition, which is the
pathologic wearing of teeth caused by involuntary action...
                                                        ↑

> Here the relative clause is in the wrong place, i.e. it is
> not next to the term it modifies. It sounds as though
> attrition is being defined, when in fact the informa-
> tion refers to abrasion.
>
> *Abrasion, which is the pathologic wearing of teeth*
> *caused by involuntary action, can be differentiated*
> *from attrition...*

Serous carcinoma is the most common subtype of epithelial
ovarian cancer and accounts for about 45% of all ovarian
cancers in the country which equates to around 30,000 cases.
                              ↑

> A comma should be inserted here to start off
> the non-essential clause.

The results described above show that NOX is activated in
both cell lines, although different dose-dependencies.
                        ↑

> Often when 'although' begins a non-essential clause,
> the following preposition or verb is mistakenly left
> out. Here 'with' has been omitted.

In the experimental group there were seven men and five
women suffered from this disease.
        ↑

> Here the relative pronoun has been left out of the clause.
> Alternatively, 'there were' could just be omitted.

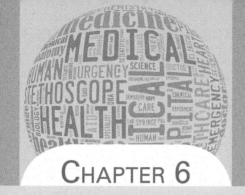

Chapter 6

Complaint F: Prefixes

Signs:
→ Inability to interpret the meaning of unfamiliar terms
→ Failing to use the correct prefix

Treatment

Prefixes are tags at the beginning of words that modify the word. Many medical terms contain prefixes and although it is not always possible to judge what particular prefix should be used, they are useful to learn as they do have specific meanings. Some relate to parts of the body such as these:

adeno- gland	**adip-** fat
angi- vessel	**brachi-** arm
cost- rib	**hepat-** liver
ment- chin	**my-** muscle
nephr- kidney	**ot-** ear
pleur- rib	**rachi-** spine
sarco- flesh/muscle	**stoma-** mouth

Some relate to position on the body:

ante- before, forward, in front of	**anti-** against
endo- inside, within	**epi-** on, outer

inter- between, among

intra- within, inside

peri- near, surrounding

post- after

pre- before

sub- under, below, beneath

trans- across, over, through

Other prefixes found in medicine are more general and are used in other disciplines and in everyday English. These prefixes relate to the presence and absence of something and strength and similarity, and they can also have positive or negative connotations.

The next time a new word is encountered, the meaning can be inferred with knowledge of these prefixes.

de–	taking something away, opposite		
dis–	reverse, opposite	**dys–**	difficult, bad, abnormal
homo–	same, alike	**hyper–**	excessive, above
in–	not, negative	**iso–**	equal, same
mal–	bad, abnormal	**mis–**	bad, wrong
non–	not, absence of	**non–**	not
poly–	many	**re–**	again, repeatedly
un–	not, opposite (not always a negative meaning)		

Recognise the correct form

Errors often occur when using the prefixes listed above as these sets of letters commonly form new words from existing ones (unlike say the prefix 'para' in 'parallel' whose root is not a word) and writers may come unstuck guessing or confusing the form. The following is a list of key terms from the medical sciences that contain these prefixes along with the associated errors.

de– decalcified   decontamination   dehydration degassing   degenerative   degraded   demotivate depolarisation   depressor   detoxify

dis– disability   discolour   discomfort   discourage   discredit disengagement   disequilibrium   disinfect   disintegrant disintegration   disinterest   disorder   displace   disprove disregard   dissimilar   dissimilarity   dissociate   distend

The following take **dys-** dysfunction dysmotility dysregulate

*They studied the effects of therapy on physical activity and quality of life in adults with a physical ~~inability~~ (**disability**)...*

inability is used for being unable to do a particular thing

*The decision to replace the socket is usually a result of ~~uncomfort~~ (**discomfort**).*

BUT/uncomfortable   ~~discomfortable~~

im– imbalance immobile immature impair impalpable impermeable implant impossible imprecise impure

*It has been reported that substance P is responsible for this ~~unbalance~~ (**imbalance**).*

in– inability inaccessible inactive inadequate incoherent inconsistent incontinent incurable indwelling ineffective ineligible inexpensive infertile inoperable insignificant insoluble instability insufficient intolerable involuntary

---

INTERVENTION   **inflammable**

Inflammable is not the negative form of flammable. They mean the same thing; however, flammable is the preferred choice and is always used on warning signs.

Some of these emollients are flammable so care was taken...

---

*The highest risk of morbidity and mortality was seen among individuals who were obese, unfit and ~~unactive~~ (**inactive**).*

*During this stage the sensors were attached by one person to avoid ~~unconsistency~~ (**inconsistency**).*

*This might explain why oxygen was ~~unaffective~~ (**ineffective**) in improving the condition.*

BUT/unaffected

*In their study, women were ~~uneligible~~ (**ineligible**) if they had any contraindication to medical abortion.*

*The changes create ~~unstability~~ (**instability**) in the gut and can lead to…*

BUT/unstable (see a–z) NOT ~~instable~~

ASSESSMENT   **inter- and intra-**

inter – between, among, during   intra – within, inside

intercellular/intracellular   intercostal   interstitial

intra-articular   intracranial   intravascular   intravenous
(not ~~intervenous~~)

mal– malabsorption   malformation   malnourished
malnutrition   malposition   malpractice   malpresentation

mis– miscarry   misdiagnose   misinform   mismatch   mistreated

*Any complaint or evidence that a patient has been ~~untreated~~ (**mistreated**) will be filed…*

'untreated' means not treated whereas mistreated means treated badly.

non– nonadherence   nonalcoholic   nonfunctioning
noninfectious   noninvasive   nonmotile   nonprescribed
nonsmoking   nonspecific   nonsterile   nonsurgical

The most likely mistake with this prefix is writing 'no' or 'not'.

*A ~~no-immune~~ (**non-immune**) antibody was used as a negative control for ~~not-specific~~ (**nonspecific**) binding.*

ASSESSMENT   **pre- and post-**

pre – before, in front of, prior to   post – behind, after

Hyphens are preferable with these prefixes.

pre-/post-operability   pre-/post-natal

pre-/post-menopausal   pre-/post-surgery

pre-existing   post-mortem   post-traumatic

---

re– reabsorption   reactive   reassess   recirculated   recollect
re-emerge   rehydrate   relapse   rematerialise   reoperate
reschedule   resuscitation

self- is always used with a hyphen.

self-harm   self-limiting   self-reported   self-management

ASSESSMENT   **super- and supra-**

super – above, on top   supra – over, outside of, beyond

suprarenal   suprasellar (NOT ~~supracellar~~)   supraventricular

superinfection   supernumerary   superovulation   supersaturation

---

un– unable   unabsorbed   unaware   unbound   uncertain
unchanged   uncommon   uncontrolled   uncooperative
unconscious   undesirable   undetected   undigested
undissolved   unexplained   unexplored   unhygienic   unlike
unmeasured   unmetabolised   unobserved   unpredictable
unprotected   unreliable   unrealistic   unreleased
unresponsiveness   unstable   unsteady   untreated

~~Dislike~~ (**Unlike**) *cellulose, glucose polymers have a branched structure
enabling them to form viscous solutions.*

'dislike' is a verb

Use them if they are available

If there is a valid and commonly used prefix (check that the prefix can be attached to that particular word if unsure) for the opposite, alternative, negative, or the repeated meaning then use it. It is always preferable to adding 'not' 'or 'again'.

*Based on this we need to ~~assess again~~ (**reassess**) the discomfort thresholds...*

These are categorised as not gastrointestinal symptoms   ✗

These are categorised as no gastrointestinal symptoms   ✗

These are categorised as nongastrointestinal symptoms   ✓

The negative past participle forms can also be used here:

*They would expect to have ~~not restricted~~ (**unrestricted**) access to the patients...*

*The ~~wrong diagnosed~~ (**misdiagnosed**) group waited only three days for this.*

Not knowing a prefix is even more apparent when the sentence appears to begin in a positive way (*This makes it...*), producing a cumbersome and awkward reading.

This makes it not a suitable method.   ✗

This makes it an unsuitable method.   ✓

Sometimes a choice can be made between a negative beginning to the sentence or a prefix indicating negation.

All other patients were not affected   ✗

No other patients were affected   ✓

All other patients were unaffected   ✓

Know when to use hyphens

It is general practice to refrain from using a hyphen after a prefix, unless the term is difficult to read.

That said, hyphens will be required for the following:

all-   self-   ex-   half-   quarter-

*One advantage is that it is **self-regulating**.*

*This increases the **half-life** of factor VIII.*

*An **all-encompassing** system is unrealistic at the current time.*

And if the word has two different meanings, a hyphen can be used to differentiate.

recover –   *This will give the patients ample time to **recover**.*

re-cover –   *It is essential to **re-cover** the equipment the next time it is moved.*

A hyphen is also used with abbreviations.

*This is in the **non-GA** group.*

Section II

Elements and data

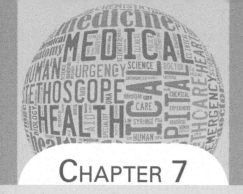

CHAPTER 7

Complaint G: Time

Signs:
→ Confusing the prepositions in time phrases
→ Not knowing when to use the singular form
→ Failing to use the correct tense

Treatment

Selecting the correct expression for time periods can be confusing. The following chart shows the general start and end points.

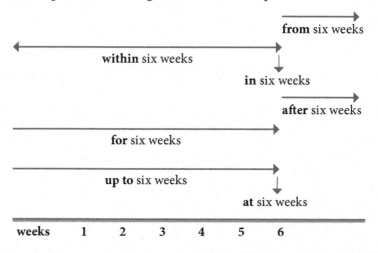

Select the correct preposition
– for/up to
These are similar but the use of 'up to' implies that something may not be as long as say six weeks. Again, use 'for' when the duration is more certain.

*This may last **up to** six weeks if untreated.*

*The participants took the medication **for** six weeks.*

– for/from
From the figure, 'for' is used to represent the entire length of time while 'from' can describe something that will begin to take place at a certain point in the future.

*This was then mixed ~~from~~ (**for**) ninety seconds.*

*But an improvement should be apparent **from** three weeks.*

– of/from
The most common error involving these two is illustrated in the following phrase:

*Within hours ~~from~~ (**of**) taking the medication…*

– within/in
These are similar but the use of 'within' implies that something may happen before the six weeks has elapsed. 'In' is used for when something will change or occur only once the six weeks are completed.

*Changes should be apparent **within** six weeks.*

*We will look at the situation again **in** six weeks.*

– within/after
'after' should be used when something is carried out once a specific length of time has elapsed.

*~~Within~~ (**After**) ten days the patients were measured again.*

If the patients need to be measured before ten days have elapsed, then 'within' can be used.

*The patients need to be measured **within** ten days of the surgery.*

– within/for

Again, a key difference between these terms is that 'for' implies that something will take place for that length of time (not shorter), whereas 'within' means a change occurs at a certain point during the course of the time period.

*We would expect to observe a difference ~~for~~ (**within**) twenty minutes.*

*They remained in the observation room **for** twenty minutes.*

– since/from

'*from*' can indicate a specific place or time as a starting point.

***From** 2018, this will be mandatory for all devices.*

Use '*from*' to also indicate the first of two specific points (with '*to*' or '*until*').

*...**from** six until seven.*

As a preposition 'since' is used to mean continuously from a certain time.

*This has been occurring **since** the parameters were changed.*

The use of '*since*' and '*from*' can therefore be contrasted by the time of the event.

*We have been studying this **since** April.*   present

*We will be analysing this data **from** October.*   future

For time-related sentences, 'since' cannot be used with the simple present tense.

*Since 2005, version 5 ~~evolves~~ (**has evolved**) to include a source list.*

It can be used with different tenses as a conjunction meaning 'as' or 'given'.

Since it is affecting consumption, we take steps to...

– until/by

Use 'until' when the activity continues up to a specific end point.

*We will continue **until** there is no more liquid in the bottle.*

Use 'by' to set a time limit for an activity or situation.

*The effects should wear off **by** 18:00.*

*The treatment will be finished ~~until~~ (**by**) the end of the week.*

Learn when to keep things singular

When discussing time periods generally (i.e. not in the methods section), remember to use the plural form for more than one minute, hour, day, week, month, year...

*The whole process could last three ~~month~~ (**months**).*

*This took place over the course of 4–5 ~~hour~~ (**hours**)*

but/ for methods write

*This was added to the sample and then incubated for **2 h**.*

When a time period is modifying a noun, it needs to be in singular form. Look at these examples:

*They also suggested a ~~ten days course~~ (**ten-day course**) of treatment.*

*There was a ~~two weeks interval~~ (**two-week interval**) between the first and second meetings.*

*This took place over a ~~four years period~~ (**four-year period**).*

Keep good time

Note the prepositions used in these time sequences:

For this we measured the mRNA levels...

> **at** the beginning   **in** the middle   **at** the end
>   ↑

> 'in the end' usually means after all or finally and describes an outcome or how something was eventually done. It is not a strict time expression.

***in** the morning   **in** the evening*

***at** noon   **at** night*

***in** the afternoon   **on** the day (of surgery)*

The samples were left ~~for~~ overnight.

in time –   Before a certain time; eventually

over time/*with* time –   Over the course of time

on time –   Punctual; at the specified time

at the same time   *at* a point *in* time

at the following time points.

*This took place ~~in~~ (**on**) different days.*

*We tested the samples ~~in~~ (**on**) the same day.*

*The patients were tested ~~in~~ (**on**) three occasions.*

Keep to the right tense
example verbs: to smoke/to stop (smoking)

SIMPLE PAST
...stopped smoking **yesterday**
...stopped smoking **last week**
...stopped smoking **earlier today**
...stopped smoking **two days ago**

SIMPLE PRESENT
...smoke **every day**
...**always** smoke
...**sometimes** smoke
...smoke **once a week**
...**never** smoke

PRESENT PERFECT
They have smoked **several times**
They have smoked **since last week**
They have smoked **recently**
They have smoked **in the last month**

PRESENT PERFECT PROGRESSIVE
They have been smoking **recently**
They have been smoking **lately**
They have been smoking **since the age of 16**
They have been smoking **this week**

*A few years ago this condition ~~has been~~ (**was**) unknown.*

*This is the first time cultured red blood cells ~~was~~ (**have been**) transfused...*

*In the past few years they ~~are~~ (**have been**) concentrating on...*

*In 2012 the obesity rates ~~have been~~ (**were**) slightly higher at...*

– time ranges

from 2010 to 2012 (2 years in total)

from 2010 through 2012 (3 years in total)

the period 2010–2012 (3 years in total)

*This was carried out ~~in~~ (**at**) regular intervals.*

*This was assessed at intervals (**of**) 1 min.*

ASSESSMENT   **–ly**

daily   *This will be carried out ~~each~~ daily*
weekly
monthly   *I used ~~month~~ (**monthly**) data.*
quarterly
yearly   *They also looked at ~~year~~ (**yearly**) projections.*

Some journals prefer the terms 'once a day/week/month' and 'twice a day/week' instead of daily, weekly, twice daily...

Eradicate certain errors

*...every 3 months for the first year, and every 6 months ~~after~~ (**thereafter**).*

*This occurred ~~after~~ 24 h (**after**) transfection.*

*A 3-fold increase was seen within 5 min ~~after~~ (**of**) the dose.*

*This is more appropriate for ~~nowaday's~~ (**today's**) Internet.*

Do not use 'nowadays' in a possessive way. It cannot be used like today's.

Nowadays, it is common to see this type of system.

---

*The ~~recent~~ (**past**) ten years have seen rapid advances in the management of...*

'past' is preferred to 'last' as the latter can mean final.

The last days are made as comfortable as possible for the sufferer.

~~Up to date~~ (**To date**), *there is no system in place to identify these patients...* ↑

"to date" is a phrase that is often used at the beginning of a sentence to mean up to now or at the present time

"up to date" is an adjective meaning current or having the latest information or style

After 60 days the treatment, we evaluated the bone regeneration...   ✗

Sixty days after the treatment, we evaluated the bone regeneration...   ✓

The evidence ~~date~~ (**dates**) *back* ~~in~~ (**to**) *1970 when Morgan and his colleagues...*

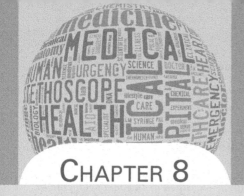

CHAPTER 8

Complaint H: People

Signs:
→ Using unsuitable terms for patients, ages and races

Treatment

For human studies there are a number of terms that should be avoided. Writers need to ensure that participants in a study are not dehumanised or come across as mere objects or simply the means by which research can achieve its objectives. When referring to patients and groups of people it should therefore be done as respectfully as possible.

Know which terms to use

The current advice is to avoid the terms in italics and employ the terms in bold instead.

case (to describe a human)   **patient**

One ~~case~~ (**patient**) who was suffering from peripheral vascular disease was particularly...

subject   **patient/participant**

A study found that there was a strong relationship between the perceived satisfaction of the ~~subjects~~ (**patients**) and nurse–patient interaction (14).

an anaemic...   **a patient with anaemia...**

*The ~~asthmatics~~ (**patients with asthma**) had the following concerns with the scheme...*

The adjective tends to be avoided then when describing patients. Naturally, they should not be directly labelled as the disease or condition either.

Therefore, these patients cannot be classified as thrombocytopenia or heparin allergy. ✗

*Therefore, these patients cannot be classified as **having** thrombocytopenia or **a** heparin allergy.* ✓

a male/female (noun)   **male/female patient** (adjective)

*We selected just one male and one female (**patient**) with severe IBS for this stage.*

or/

We selected just one man and one woman with severe IBS for this stage.

But for animals male and female can be used as nouns.

From the ten fisher rats we chose two males and two females and fed them...

– gender and pronouns

To avoid gender bias the plural pronoun 'they' is increasingly being employed to represent the third person singular. 'They' is also used when the gender is unknown.

*The researcher can restart the process if **they** feel the conditions have changed significantly.*

Of course, if a particular individual is being described then a gender-specific pronoun is fine.

*The physiotherapist was given the necessary information before **he** entered the room.*

'It' or 'its' should not be used as a replacement for 'he/she' when referring to a person. (see also a–z *it*)

*The participant can also review this and even withdraw ~~its~~ (**their**) consent...*

*When the machine encounters a problem **it** will...*

– 'human'

When mentioning humans in a general sense use the plural form.

*~~Human is~~ (**Humans are**) affected by four main types of the disease.*

*This can protect ~~human~~ (**humans**) against many parasites.*

And the term is always plural in the phrase 'in humans'.

*Influenza B only occurs in ~~human~~ (**humans**).*

Never use a definite article.

It became prevalent in ~~the~~ humans towards the end of the nineteenth century.

You can write 'a human' if you are making a contrast with an animal.

*Animals would react quickly in this situation. **A human** however would not be able to detect such a change.*

And if 'human' precedes another noun it acts like an adjective and takes the singular form.

*This has increased because of ~~humans~~ (**human**) activity.*

*There are ~~humans~~ (**human**) factors involved that exacerbate the problem.*

– age

Mistakes occur when discussing the ages of patients and participants.

—Years old/years of age

When mentioning someone's age use this form.

The first participant was 17 years of age.

This is often preferred to '17 years old' (year-old is fine as an adjective in a compound '*a ten-year-old boy*'). It is unnecessary to use both 'aged' and 'years old/years of age'.

We concentrated on those aged between 50 and 69 ~~years old~~.

But retain the unit of age for children as they could be months or years.

*This was mainly introduced for those aged 5 (**months/years**) and older.*

age – noun and verb

aged – adjective and past tense of the verb 'to age'.

*It was important that their ~~aged~~ (**age**) was not below eighteen.*

CASE REPORT: MIDDLE AGE

As a general rule, middle age should only be used before 'of' or 'in' to represent the idea of being in the middle of life.

He was in middle age.
He was of middle age.

'Middle-aged' describes the general age of someone but it is quite vague for the reader.

*Sixty **middle-aged** men were selected from rural areas.*

If the cohort is middle-aged, be specific and state the age ranges.

ASSESSMENT   **age ranges**

A general age classification to follow is

newborn – up to 1 month   infant – 1 month to 1 year
child – 2–12 years of age   teenage – 13–19 years of age
adolescent – 13–17 years of age   adult – 18 and over
elderly – 65 years of age and over

---

*~~In~~ (**At**) this age there is a strong desire to...*

*Each ~~ages~~ (**age**) category was also assigned a...*

*The 60-~~days~~ (**day**)-old rats were then transferred to...*

*This may also strengthen the motivation in ~~old~~ (**elderly**) patients who have...*

– nationality and countries

In medicine, nationality may not always be a suitable category on which to base a study or trial given the many racial variations within a nation. But some studies may achieve useful results from country of birth or residence, in which case note the difference between the noun form and the adjective.

Name of area	Adjective for people
USA/US	American(s)
Germany	German(s)
Spain	Spanish
Italy	Italian(s)
France	French
UK	British (technically Great Britain does not include Northern Ireland. However, 'British' is accepted as an adjective for 'Britain', which is a shortened form of the United Kingdom of Great Britain and Northern Ireland, so it is generally used for all nations except the Republic of Ireland. Does the study cover the whole of the UK or can you be more specific?)
England	English
Scotland	Scottish
Wales	Welsh
Northern Ireland	Northern Irish
Ireland	Irish
China	Chinese
Japan	Japanese
Europe	European(s)

*The study took place in ~~German~~ (**Germany**) and France...*

*Twenty ~~China~~ (**Chinese**) participants were selected from...*

INTERVENTION   adjective order

In the standard order of adjectives, age comes before nationality.

*They studied the ~~Hispanic elderly~~ **elderly Hispanic** population to discover whether...*

The patient was a Japanese 60-year-old man with no prior history of... ✗

The patient was a 60-year-old Japanese man with no prior history of... ✓

CASE REPORT: RACE

Be as clear as possible about the ancestry of the participants. 'Twenty Canadian participants' could comprise participants of Asian descent and Eurasian descent, which may be relevant when drawing conclusions.

We recruited twenty participants from Canada, three of which were of African American descent, two had Chinese ancestry and the other fifteen were white.

Of course if the label is based on country of birth or years based in the country this needs to be clarified.

It should be noted that Hispanic and Latino are terms of ethnicity and not race. General race categories are American Indian, Alaska Native, Asian, Black/African American, Native Hawaiian/Pacific Islander, White.

Note also that some journals and institutes prefer 'white' to 'Caucasian' and with no capital letter.

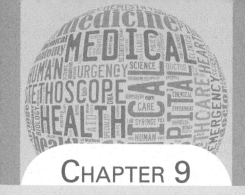

CHAPTER 9

Complaint I: Numbers and stats

Signs:
→ Misusing numbers and percentages
→ Confusing statistical terms

Treatment

Most researchers rely heavily on numbers and stats to justify their arguments and theories, and papers are judged by the accuracy and importance of the figures that are provided. With so many hours spent identifying patterns and implications in a study's results, it would be a shame for the basic formatting and grammar to let the researcher and the paper down.

INTERVENTION			number errors
~~thirtey~~	thirty (30)	~~fourty~~	forty (40)
~~fifthty~~	fifty (50)	~~eightey~~	eighty (80)
~~eight one~~	eighty one (81)	~~two hundreds~~	two hundred (200)

Learn a few conventions

Using a number and a unit to modify a scale should be avoided where possible and rewritten with an 'of' phrase.

This resulted in a 6 kg weight increase. ✗

This resulted in a weight increase of 6 kg. ✓

Numbers (not words) should always be used with units.

An incision was made of approximately ~~ten~~ (10) mm.

If the number is not linked to a unit then spell the word out for numbers below 11, unless they are included in a range.

Only ~~5~~ (five) metabolites were found in the faecal slurries of the healthy control group...

An ideal range would be from ~~eight to sixteen~~ (8 to 16).

If another number precedes a unit number then spell out the number even if it is above 11.

Afterwards, ~~12~~ (twelve) 500 mL vessels were procured and filled with...

Otherwise use numbers for 11 and above unless they begin a sentence.

The total number of cases was ~~three hundred and seventy nine~~ (379).

***Twenty five** items from the original **50** were selected.*

A leading zero is preferred for decimals.

~~.045~~   **0.045**

Commas are generally preferred to spaces.

~~6 000 000~~   **6,000,000**

Organise the units of measure

Some schools and journals prefer SI whereas others prescribe conventional units. There is merit in stating both.

Following this 7 fl oz (210 mL) was prepared using...

Providing a conversion is also good practice.

The values are as follows: Red blood cells, $2.6 \times 10^6/\mu L$ (to convert to $\times 10^{12}/L$, multiply by 1.0)...

Units that are not linked to numbers should be spelled out.

*Naturally this will also be measured in ~~g/L~~ (**grams per litre**).*

If a number and unit begin a sentence then the unit should be written in full.

*Fifty ~~mg~~ (**milligrams**) is a sufficient dose but 100 mg....*

Units of measure should not be pluralised and they take singular verbs.

*In brief, ~~2.5 mLs~~ (**2.5 mL**) of reagent was added to ~~200 µLs~~ (**200 µL**) of water... the absorbance at ~~540 nms~~ (**540 nm**) was measured after ~~5 mins~~ (**5 min**)...*

Informal measures will require plurals for more than one.

*Three ~~drop~~ (**drops**) were added daily for 25 ~~day~~ (**days**)...*

For concentrations the 'of' is normally omitted.

Absorbance was calculated using 50–800 µg/mL ~~of~~ gallic acid...

The unit should be placed next to the number with no spaces in between.

*In the third experiment, ~~80 %~~ (**80%**) was retained when stored at ~~4.5 °C~~ (**4.5°C**)...*

Know where to position the number

Numbers go after the sequence word (first, next, last) and before the modifying word.

*The **next three tasks** were presented to the subjects as...*

*These are the **two main contributions** of this study.*

*We facilitated **twenty physiotherapy sessions** that...*

Additional three tests were carried out...   ✗

Three additional tests were carried out...   ✓

Use percentages correctly

Use '%' and not 'percent/percentage/percentages' with numbers.

*The variation is slightly higher than 80 ~~percentage~~ (**%**)...*

But if it is the first word of the sentence, spell out the number and use 'percent'.

***Ten percent** is an appropriate starting point...*

You can write 'percentages' when it is not connected to a number.

*The **percentages** of positive cells analysed by confocal microscopy were...*

Remember the 'of' phrase in this construction.

*28% (**of the**) damage occurred after the fall.*

And do not use a comma as a decimal point.

*~~98,9%~~ (**98.9%**)*

The noun following the percentage should determine whether the verb is singular or plural.

*20% of the patients **are** eligible to proceed to the next phase.*

*25% of the training **was** supervised.*

And the noun will determine the use of fewer and less.

***Fewer** than 20% of the patients are eligible…*

***Less** than 25% of the training was supervised.*

Recognise when to use rank

Ordinal numbers are used for order and rank. Do not use an ordinal to represent a quantity.

*~~Fourteenth~~ (**Fourteen**) sets of fermentations were performed using samples from…*

Here, an ordinal is required but a regular number has been used by mistake.

*A study reported it as the ~~eight~~ (**eighth**) most common cause of _____ in the US.*

For a series of ordinals use the numeric shorthand.

Next we will look at the third, sixth and ninth weeks.   ✗

Next we will look at the 3rd, 6th and 9th weeks.   ✓

INTERVENTION   **ordinal numbers**

These are the most commonly misused and misspelled ordinals:

(~~3th~~)   third (3rd)   ~~forth~~   fourth (4th)

~~twelth~~   ~~twelf~~   twelfth (12th)

~~thirtenth~~   thirteenth (13th)

~~fourtieth~~ ~~fortyth~~   fortieth (40th)

Work with ranges

A range must consist of more than one number or value.

The age range was 45 years.   ✗

Do not mix from/to with hyphens.

The prevalence in Canada varies from 10%–15%   ✗

The prevalence in Canada varies from 10% to 15%   ✓

Units of measure should ideally be used with both numbers.

This solution varied from 64 to 72°C during the...   ✗

This solution varied from 64°C to 72°C during the...   ✓

*The interviews will last ~~in the range of~~ (**for**) 30 minutes.*

*The interviews **ranged from** 30 to 45 minutes.*

*The number of participants was between 20 ~~or~~ (**and**) 40.*

*This was then increased from 3.5 ~~and~~ (**to**) 6.5.*

*The ratio is between ~~0 to 1~~ (**0 and 1**).*

*The levels will vary from ~~0 and 5~~ (**0 to 5**).*

*This is likely to be ~~on~~ (**in**) the range of 70 to 150.*

Note the common mistakes

*The dialysis tube was placed in a ~~twoL~~ (**2 L**) beaker and incubated for ~~6hrs~~ (**6 h**).*

*In this study, pain intensity is measured on ~~a~~ (**an**) 11-point, ~~0 to ten~~ (**0–10**) numerical rating scale (NRS). For NRS, a ~~10%~~ (**10%**) to 20% (1.1 ~~and~~ (**to**) 2.2 point) decrease is considered clinically important.*

The threshold is equals to the noise level /ERB$_N$.   ✗

The threshold equals to the noise level /ERB$_N$.   ✗

*The threshold **is equal to** the noise level /ERB$_N$.*   ✓

*The threshold **equals** the noise level /ERB$_N$.*   ✓

> **INTERVENTION**   fractions
>
> ~~two third~~ two thirds   ~~one quarters~~ one quarter
> ~~third quarters~~ three quarters

*We compare this to the three ~~type~~ (**types**) of care...*

We investigated the relationship between these biomarkers and all four ~~numbers of~~ equations.

Many ~~numbers of~~ clinical trials have been conducted to confirm the relationship between...

*The ~~amount of~~ (**number of**) adherent cells had reduced...*

> Use 'number of' for plural and 'amount of' for uncountable nouns. *The amount of evidence...*

This will not be measured if it is below ~~than~~ two.

The participant must then select a number over ~~than~~ five.

> **CASE REPORT: TWICE/DOUBLE**
>
> Twice can only be used as an adverb; double can be used as a noun, adjective, adverb and verb. There is some overlap in meaning but as a guideline use 'twice' to mean 'two times' and for comparison alongside 'as'. Use double for expressing quantity, specifically for multiplying by two or as much again in size, strength or number.
>
> *In this scenario the dose would be ~~twice~~ (**doubled**).*
>
> *There were ~~double as~~ (**twice as**) many withdrawals...*

Check the stats

When it comes to mistakes made using statistical terms, the usual suspects can be found in the box below:

1. Do not confuse the analysis of variance with the analysis of covariance. Neither term requires an explanation on first use. *A 2 × 2 **ANOVA** (~~analysis of variance~~) examined the effects...*

2. The intervals are confidence intervals not confident.

3. Data is continuous not continues.

4. An observed continuous variable is the covariate not the covariant.

5. It is Cronbach not Chronbach.

6. The plural is degrees of freedom not degree of freedoms.

7. A common typo is liner.

8. You can have regression to the mean but not regression with the mean. Ensure that mean is not pluralised when used as a modifier. *We looked at the means (mean) operating time. The means (mean) age of the participants was...*

> *Statistical terms misused*
>
> 1. ANOVA/ANCOVA
> 2. confidence
> 3. continuous
> 4. covariate
> 5. Cronbach's alpha
> 6. degrees of freedom
> 7. linear
> 8. mean
> 9. odds ratio
> 10. parametric
> 11. Student t-test

9. It is an odds ratio not an odd ratio.

10. The methods and tests are parametric and nonparametric. Hyphens are not required. *Both of the nonparameter (**nonparametric**) methods were used because they could effectively deal with the small sample sizes.*

11. Most guidelines advise using an initial capital for Student, using italics for *t* and then hyphenating: Student *t*-test.

– significance

When discussing the significance of something in statistical terms, the adverb 'statistically' is not necessary.

All the comparisons were considered statistically significant when $p < 0.05$.

Stop to consider whether the noun or adjective is required.

*There was no significance (**significant**) difference in the number or characteristics.*

*This makes it difficult to detect small but potentially significance (**significant**) differences across groups.*

*This increase still failed to reach significant (**significance**).*

*The reviewer suggested using a two-sided test with a significant (**significance**) level of 5%.*

– insignificant vs. nonsignificant

Use nonsignificant or not significant for statistics. Even if the result is not significant it may not be insignificant to you or your readers.

– use tables

Effective use of tables will make the data manageable and ensure the results section is concise and easy to read and easy to follow.

> Short title that sufficiently explains the table. Table should be numbered and referred to in the text as near to the table as possible.

Table 5. Prevalence of identified disorders stratified by weight

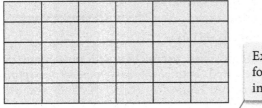

> Explanation at the foot of the table not in the title

Data expressed as Mean S.D. Figures in parentheses are number of subjects. BP: Blood pressure; LDL: Low-density lipoprotein...*P < 0.01, **P < 0.001...

> Data explained, abbreviations defined and statistical values outlined

Note the common errors made when referring to tables and figures.

> Articles are not used when the figure or table is numbered.

From ~~the~~ Table 3 it is clear that...

The thresholds of the control group are ~~below shown~~ (**shown below**).

The ~~below table~~ (**table below**) demonstrates the relationship between...

'below' should not be used as an adjective. Note that above can be used as an adjective: 'above table'/'table above'

These operations are shown ~~at~~ (**in**) Figure 11.

Use 'in' for tables and figures not 'on' or 'at'.

SECTION III

Style

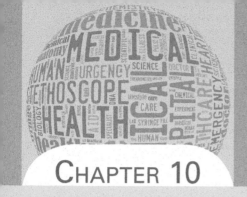

CHAPTER 10

Complaint J: Tense

> Signs:
> → Having trouble forming tenses
> → Inability to select the correct tense

Treatment

Tenses are used to mark the time of an action or an event.

Initially, we can split the tenses into present, past and future: (verb – to test)

present: *It* **tests** *a number of cell lines linked to the...*

past: *They* **tested** *a number of cell lines linked to the...*

future: *We* **will test** *a number of cell lines linked to the...*

Of course not all sentences contain a pronoun, and sometimes this is forgotten when learning verb conjugation and lists of 'I test, he tests, they test...' The key to effective writing and to reducing mistakes is applying the knowledge to your own writing. So here are examples of the three tenses without those traditional pronouns.

One study **tests** *whether this has a long-term effect as well.*

Morgan (2009) **tested** *this approach and discovered that...*

*This third activity **will test** the ability of the compounds to reduce...*

In the simple future tense the verb form stays the same. We use 'will' along with the normal or dictionary form of the verb.

The examples above are all in the simple aspect. There are other aspects that assist the writer in being more exact about the time of an event or action.

Learn the aspects
– perfect

*The technique **has changed** with technological advances...*

↑

> **present perfect:** Action that begins in the past but continues into the present or the effect continues.

*A 25-year-old patient revealed that a mole **had changed** when they visited a second time.*

↑

> **past perfect:** Action in the past and completed before another action.

*The virus **will have changed** by the time the product is ready.*

↑

> **future perfect:** Action that will have been completed at a specific time in the future.

– progressive

*This **is changing** the way that drugs are prescribed...*

↑

> **present progressive:** Action happening at the moment or fixed in the near future.

*One third stated **they were changing** their medication...*

↑

> **past progressive:** Action that was happening at some point in the past.

*They **will be changing** the labelling of their products...*

↑

> **future progressive:** Action that will be happening at some point in the future.

There is also a perfect progressive form:

present perfect progressive: *It has been changing*

past perfect progressive: *It had been changing*

future perfect progressive: *It will have been changing*

CASE REPORT: PAST PERFECT TENSE

The past perfect can be overused and in fact is quite limited. It is only used to refer to an event in the past if another event beginning in the past is also being mentioned. When describing one event that took place in the past, just use the past tense.

At this stage we changed the growth conditions of the bacteria.

one event – simple past

They had finished the interviews when the hospital manager arrived.

two events – past perfect

Know when to change tenses

As a general rule tenses should remain consistent in a sentence or paragraph, unless the time of the action being described alters or the viewpoint of the author/researcher changes.

*We **obtained** an SDP in the fixed transmit sequence case and **devised** new algorithms to synthesise the transmit sequences.*

But there are many occasions where the tense can be changed in a sentence, especially when the main verb is in the present or future tense. If the main verb is in these tenses, the subordinate verbs can be in any tense.

*Our findings **demonstrate** that this approach **inhibited** the targeted subgroups.*

An example of a subtle shift in tense is when the sentence begins with a time expression (such as *when, before, after, if, unless*); here, the first part of the clause is in the present tense and the second in the future.

present		future

When they increase their intake   *gastrointestinal symptoms will reappear.*

Confusion arises when the writer attempts to follow guidelines asking for, say, the literature review to be written in the past tense. The temptation is then to write every verb in the past tense.

*In general terms, colonisation of the gut by this type of bacteria was (**is**) essential to human health. Morgan **analysed** three types of...* ↑   ↑

Using the past tense for the literature review means that reporting verbs and any particular experiments or research are written and explained in the past tense. In the example above a well-known fact is stated, so the verb should be in the present tense. If something is still true today or is a current event the past tense is inappropriate. Even if a particular tense is to be favoured, each verb should still be assessed for appropriate usage.

Verbals can take a different tense to the main verb in the past and perfect forms. Here the action takes place before that of the main verb:

*Male patients **showing** increased activity in regions involved in pain inhibition **supported** our argument.*

– using the appropriate tense

When reporting results or detailing methods or events, the past tense is usually used.

*As previously reported, Morgan **conducted** experiments to test this theory (12, 14).*

The present tense is useful to show that the method or finding is relevant and accepted, because it can project a sense of significance or importance.

*Interestingly, they **reveal** that it **is** because these factors have a smaller influence.*

Key points in the analysis (results) of your own tests can also work well in the present tense.

*The results of our analysis **indicate** that the cause is primarily environmental.*

As noted earlier, for a well-known fact or result that is generally accepted in the field the present tense is used – regardless of the tenses around it or its location in the work (i.e. conclusion, introduction, methods section).

A palpitation is an increased awareness of the heartbeat.

The disease progresses quickly to cardiac failure and is often fatal.

The present perfect (and present perfect progressive) is used to describe the general trend in a specific research area. It usually introduces the current situation before specific studies are explored in more detail or your own methods are revealed.

*The studies **have focused** on the inter-individual variation in relation to ethnicity, ageing, and colonic health status.*

*Researchers **have been studying** these breast cancer markers…*

When summarising or concluding, the past tense is the clear choice. A common mistake is to use the present tense when referring to earlier sections of a paper.

*The previous chapter ~~looks~~ (**looked**) at interventions aimed at weight gain prevention and ~~assess~~ (**assessed**) three schemes designed to…*

When referring to tables and diagrams that follow, it is logical to use the present tense and not the past.

...this ~~was shown~~ (is shown) in the following table:

Plan for the future

One ambiguity is that we do not always have to use the future tense to discuss future plans or events.

We know that 'will' is used before the verb to discuss future events generally.

*This evaluation **will** be carried out by studying the correlation between...*

But when we know about the future we can actually use the present tense. Here something has been arranged and the present tense is used.

*They **have** further consultations next week.*

Future plans can also be mentioned in the present progressive.

*They **are planning** to add another group to the trial.*

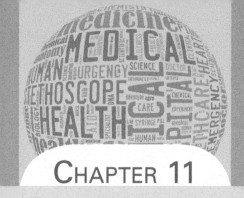

Chapter 11

Complaint K: Verbs and voice

Signs:
→ Failing to understand the relationship between active and passive writing
→ Using weak verb forms
→ Using the wrong verbs for reporting and claiming

Treatment

Medical papers are generally written with a procedure-driven narrative with the writer using a passive voice for the most part. That said, the active voice is beginning to find favour with both editors and authors as a more dynamic way of presenting and describing research. An appreciation of the structural differences and the suitability of both active and passive voice will help you to make the right choices for your own paper.

There are two voices in English, active and passive. The subject performs the action in a sentence with an active voice.

We analyse the discomfort thresholds to confirm the lack of a relationship between...

The word order can be altered in some situations to make the sentence passive. The subject then goes from performing the action to being acted upon by the verb.

The discomfort thresholds were analysed to confirm the lack of a relationship between...

In the passive voice a form of 'to be' (in this case 'were') is used and comes before the past participle (analysed).

ASSESSMENT   **pronouns**

Pronouns are removed when changing from active to passive.

We note an error here.   *An error was noted here.*

They used a pie chart to...   *A pie chart was used...*

Even if the active sentence is in the present tense, the passive sentence will still use the past participle.

Understand the relationship between voice and tense

When changing a sentence from active to passive the tense does not change. If the active sentence was in the past tense then use this for the passive sentence as well.

We collected cells in an Eppendorf tube and spun them at 1500 rpm for 90 sec...

Cells were collected in an Eppendorf tube and spun at...

Because the –ed form is generally associated with the past tense, errors can occur when the passive is used for a present action.

*The UV light transmission is record (**recorded**) by the camera...*

In the active voice the sentence would read:

The camera records the UV light transmission

– the verb 'to be'

Note which form of the verb 'to be' to use for the passive voice in the progressive and perfect tenses.

progressive tense:
(add 'being')

The company is changing the product name.

The product name is being changed (by the company).

perfect tense:
(add 'been')

The company has changed the product name...

The product name has been changed...

CASE REPORT: A PASSIVE PROBLEM

Using the passive voice can sometimes lead to a subject that is too complex and too far away from the verb.

A solution for reducing workload and ensuring patient data is updated regularly and by the relevant staff has been found.   ✗

A solution has been found for reducing workload and...   ✓

Appreciate the merits of both voices

The **passive** voice is employed by many medical writers because it is effective at describing methods and procedures and adds formality to the text. It is also used by writers when they wish to remain neutral. It takes the focus off the subject or the person carrying out the action and puts attention onto the way something has been carried out. This is why passive voice is often employed in abstracts.

A prospective, open-labelled clinical trial was undertaken...severity was graded by...serum was administered as an...nonparametric tests were used in...clinical recovery was noted...

The **active** voice is employed to make the sentences more appealing to the reader and for the writer to get a point across in a direct and clear way. Another effect is that the subject takes responsibility for the action.

The researchers ended the study too quickly...

In the passive version the researchers do not have to be mentioned, so the blame can be just implied.

The study was ended too quickly (by the researchers).

The above example shows the active voice being used to criticise, but equally it can be employed to promote and emphasise a finding or a method.

Consequently, Morgan failed to identify the nature of the hypersensitivity (9). **We *include*** *a control group of healthy volunteers…*

> Contrast with the weaker passive version:
>
> *Consequently, Morgan failed to identify the nature of the hypersensitivity (9). A control group of healthy volunteers was included in our study…*

The researcher can therefore demonstrate how their work improves on the work of others and perhaps how innovative and unique the research is by using active sentences. The passive voice tends to present the methods and procedures as normal or standard ones without really promoting what is being done.

The main danger with the active voice is the tendency for every sentence to start with a personal pronoun. This can be avoided by combining active sentences with passive ones.

We therefore ensured that the surfactant did not exceed the CMC concentration. The procedure was carried out over…

> Rather than 'We carried out the procedure…'

The passive voice still implies something being done by somebody. In fact the inclusion of the verb 'to be' (in the second example below) allows the writer to describe an action the researcher has directly carried out.

*The level **increased** significantly in European participants on the high-polyphenol diet.*

(this describes the result; the event happens independently)

*To investigate this, the number of types **was increased** to four.*

(this describes something that the researcher actively changed. '*The number of types increased to four*' sounds as if it happened on its own without the researcher's influence).

– restrictions on the passive voice

Only sentences with a direct object can change voices. In other words, only verbs that are transitive (those that take objects) can be reworked into the passive form.

*We **made an error** on the second questionnaire...*	active
An error was made on the second questionnaire.	passive

> Note: *The doctor arrived at 6pm.   At 6pm the doctor arrived.*
>
> This is not an example of active and passive. The prepositional phrase has just been moved to the beginning of the sentence.

CASE REPORT: CONSIST, CONTAIN

These two verbs cannot be used with the verb 'to be' in a passive type construction.

The survey consists of 15 items on a dichotomised scale. ✓

The survey is consisted of 15 items on a dichotomised scale. ✗

This fruit contains a high antioxidant level. ✓

A high antioxidant level is contained by this fruit. ✗

Sentences with the auxiliary verb 'to have' as the main verb cannot be transformed into passive either.

The administrators had a different role.

~~A different role was had by the administrators.~~

Be aware of nominalisation

Nominalisation occurs when a verb (or adjective) is replaced by the noun form.

investigate – verb   investigation – noun

We investigated human skin fibroblasts...

An investigation was carried out on human skin fibroblasts...

The first sentence is concise and takes only two words (*we investigated*) to inform the reader that there was an investigation. The second sentence takes six words (*an investigation was carried out on*) to convey the same information.

We made an evaluation of these self-reporting methods. ✗

We evaluated these self-reporting methods. ✓

Our results were found to be in agreement with (9) and (13). ✗

Our results agreed with (9) and (13). ✓

CASE REPORT: NOMINALISITIS

Nominalisation produces phrases that add very little to a sentence. By omitting the unnecessary terms, the sentence can be almost halved in size.

The first step will be to conduct an evaluation of the whole study design.

First, we will evaluate the whole study design.

Instead of using 'there is/are' or 'there was/were', simply bring the subject back alongside a verb. This can also cut out other unnecessary phrases.

There were six problems in relation to the initial scheme.

The initial scheme had six problems.

But using nouns in this way should not be avoided altogether. It can add variety to the sentences and prevent repetition and can also provide a link to a previous idea or action. Like the variety achieved by using a mix of active and passive, verb and noun phrases can be incorporated for a similar effect.

We discussed *the various options available to the patients individually and in groups.* ***A discussion of*** *our own research aims also took place to ensure that...*

Understand that verbs can take on strong and weak properties

Once a verb has been chosen it can take on different degrees of strength depending on whether it is used actively, passively, as a verbal or nominalised. The stronger the verb form, the clearer and more dynamic the sentence.

> *If we extract the data...*   STRONG
>
> *If data are extracted...*
>
> *With extracted data...*
>
> *With extraction of data...*   WEAK

Verbs can be weakened even more by hesitant phrases.

This allows the patients more freedom to choose their course.

*This **seems to** allow the patients more freedom to choose...*

*This **might** allow the patients more freedom to choose...*

Know which verbs should be used for claims

Certain verbs are used for stating your ideas or other people's ideas and for evaluating methods and findings. These claims can be graded for strength based on the verb chosen.

Strong claim – confirm, convince, demonstrate, determine, find, know, prove, show

*We have **demonstrated** that an abnormal reading at this stage is a clear indicator of hearing loss.*

Weak/limited claim – assume, doubt, estimate, imagine, imply (see a–z), indicate, infer (see a–z *imply*), interpret, perceive, predict, presume, speculate, suggest, suppose, suspect

*Therefore, it is **assumed** that information obtained from our test can assist the clinician in providing the patient with...*

Know which verbs should be used for reporting

Certain verbs are also used for reporting other people's studies and ideas. These verbs can be used to show that a researcher has a positive or negative stance, is evaluating or contrasting something, or that they believe strongly about something.

The researcher has a strong opinion

Morgan claims/declares/maintains...

The researcher gives guidance or an opinion

Morgan proposes/recommends/predicts/projects/suggests…

The researcher does not believe in something

Morgan denies/questions/refutes/rejects…

The researcher looks closely at something

Morgan analyses/focuses/theorises…

The researcher uncovers something

Morgan discovers/finds/learns/reveals (see a–z)

ASSESSMENT   **that**

Note the relationship between the reporting verb and 'that'. 'That' after a reporting verb may mean the sentence requires a further part.

The study evaluated ~~that~~ the initial phase of the scheme.

The study revealed that the initial phase of the scheme was delayed because of…

Morgan also demonstrated that an increase in the number of enteroendocrine cells will lead to…

Technically the use of 'that' is optional here, but if it is omitted the reader may be expecting the sentence to finish earlier (as below) so it should be retained for clarity.

Morgan also demonstrated an increase in the number of enteroendocrine cells.

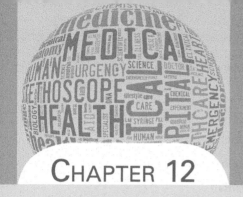

CHAPTER 12

Complaint L: Clarity and character

> Signs:
> → Writing inefficiently and without focus
> → Using the wrong style and vocabulary

Treatment

When writing a medical paper the focus should be on communicating your ideas in the most effective way possible. Although identifying unnecessary phrases and eliminating wordiness in your work can be a challenge, there are some terms you should reject immediately and others that can be efficiently modified.

Avoid redundant and unnecessary terms

Improve the quality of your writing straight away by removing the unnecessary words from these terms.

brief in duration   **brief**

The initial discussion was brief ~~in duration~~.

still continues   **continues**

This ~~still~~ continues to have an effect...

evolve over time   **evolve**

The microbiota evolves ~~over time~~ until adulthood when...

few in number   **few**

There were also minor cases but these were few ~~in number~~.

new innovation   **innovation**

It is ~~a new~~ (an) innovation that has allowed...

large/small in size   **large/small**

These osseous lesions were large ~~in size~~ so we...

may possibly   **may**

This may ~~possibly~~ lead to further complications...

brand new   **new**

This is a ~~brand~~ new approach to sourcing phytochemicals...

proceed forward   **proceed** (see also a–z)

Dermatologists can then proceed ~~forward~~ with an examination of...

continue to remain   **remain** (see also a–z)

This should ~~continue to~~ remain the situation throughout the testing phase.

return back   **return**

It meant a return ~~back~~ to the old system of handling patient data.

~~very~~ critical	**critical**	
~~very~~ crucial	**crucial**	These are strong adjectives that require no emphasis.
~~very~~ necessary	**necessary**	

A few verbs are mistaken for phrasal verbs and given an unnecessary particle.

consider ~~about~~ **consider**   discuss ~~about~~ **discuss**

increases ~~up~~ **increases**   reduces ~~down~~ **reduces**

– use acronyms and abbreviations effectively

When using acronyms and abbreviations, first define them in full and then refer to them each time in the abbreviated form.

They assessed whether this would affect physical activity levels and the number of binge eating episodes. Although behavioural therapy can be beneficial for reducing binge eating episodes (BEE), it does not necessarily lead to weight loss. ✗

They assessed whether this would affect physical activity levels and the number of binge eating episodes (BEE). Although behavioural therapy can be beneficial for reducing BEE, it does not necessarily lead to weight loss. ✓

It is important to shorten terms and utilise pronouns when an abbreviation is not available. This seems obvious enough but it is surprising how much repetition occurs in writing.

This section presents an upper limb multibody model that uses subject-specific information. The ~~upper limb multibody~~ model…

*A bone morphogenetic protein has been purified and its cDNA obtained. ~~The bone morphogenetic protein~~ (**This protein**) has the ability to induce bone when implanted…*

*Using this app helps staff decide which jobs ~~the staff~~ (**they**) should prioritise…*

And when an abbreviation is available and has already been introduced, there is no need to keep reminding the reader.

Measuring by PGV (which stands for proximal gastric volume)…

The gastric area is measured by PGV, for proximal gastric volume, and then…

Make sure to prioritise the subject

It is always good practice to place the most important point at the beginning of the sentence. Note the position of the subject here:

For typing the Rh blood group and testing the six reagents for different alleles, we used a positive and a negative control. ✗

We used a positive and a negative control for typing the Rh blood group and testing the reagents for different alleles. ✓

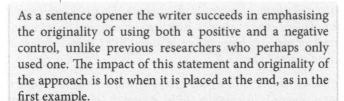

As a sentence opener the writer succeeds in emphasising the originality of using both a positive and a negative control, unlike previous researchers who perhaps only used one. The impact of this statement and originality of the approach is lost when it is placed at the end, as in the first example.

Eliminate most conjunctives

Conjunctive adverbs (furthermore, however, meanwhile...) should be used sparingly. Compare the systematic use of adverbs as clause starters in the first passage with their prudent absence in the second.

However, a frequently occurring side effect is neuropsychiatric and cognitive impairment. Indeed, a postmortem study found that long term treatment with anticholinergic drugs in patients with Parkinson's disease promotes the formation of β-amyloidosis in the brain. Additionally it promotes senile plaque in the brain, which contributes to Alzheimer-type pathology. Moreover, this finding is especially true for elderly patients (aged over 70 in this study) (8).

A frequently occurring side effect is neuropsychiatric and cognitive impairment. A postmortem study found that long term treatment with anticholinergic drugs in patients with Parkinson's disease promotes the formation of β-amyloidosis and senile plaque in the brain, which contribute to Alzheimer-type pathology especially in elderly patients (aged over 70 in this study) (8).

INTERVENTION   **such as, including**

When listing every single factor or option these two terms are redundant.

We address the four symptoms ~~such as~~: *Early satiation, epigastric pain, epigastric fullness and epigastric burning.*

The five predominant types ~~include~~ *(are) bacteroides, bifidobacteria, eubacteria, streptococci and lactobacilli.*

Keep the verbs parallel

It is always pleasing to read a run of verbs in the same clause or sentence, especially when they all have the same form. This parallel structure is demonstrated here:

*The cream was effective in **reducing** the redness, **relieving** the urge to itch and **improving** the appearance of the skin.*

No guidelines have been set for cleaning and disinfection of anaesthesia-related equipment.   ✗

No guidelines have been set for cleaning and disinfecting anaesthesia-related equipment.   ✓

The following objectives were set:

1) *To evaluate their psychosocial well-being*
2) *Providing insights into the nature of their QoL*
3) *Assess the agreement between formal caregivers and family members*

↑

Parallel structure is essential when compiling lists. Here the writer has a few options, but changing them all into the infinitive form or the base form is recommended.

1) (to) evaluate their...
2) (to) provide insights...
3) (to) assess the...

Retain the abstract style in the main body

There are some rules and regulations used for abstracts that can also be adopted in the main text to ensure that the writing is concise and focused.

No repetition of statements – There is not enough room in an abstract to repeat sentences or summarise at the beginning and the end. This should be adopted in the actual work as well. All too often the introductory statements reappear word for word in the chapter summary (albeit in a different tense) and in the main conclusion like this:

We will begin by analysing the effectiveness of the patient-oriented approach for the prescription of dialysis modalities, which aims to minimise common dialysis complications.

This chapter has analysed the effectiveness of the patient-oriented approach for the...

Having analysed the effectiveness of the patient-oriented approach for the...

Here is a typical example of a writer repeating the last point in the next sentence.

The number of people classified as obese has risen dramatically in the past 30 years. Human genes on the other hand have changed relatively little in recent times ~~compared with the number of people classified as obese in the past thirty years~~. *This increase in obesity cannot therefore be attributed to genetic factors but instead...*

No meaningless phrases or preliminary statements – Abstracts have to get to the point as quickly as possible. This should be applied to the main work as well. Every time you begin to introduce something or conclude something, think about whether it is actually necessary.

In the first section, procedures for sample size calculation, sampling and subject recruitment, data collection, and data analysis for the quasi-experimental design are explained; in the second section, the same issues for the descriptive qualitative study are discussed. In both sections, alternative approaches considered at each stage are also discussed and the choices made are justified.

This paragraph is unnecessary as the areas covered are mainstream and require no introduction or explanation. Relevant subheadings will provide the reader with everything they need.

~~A discussion of the treatments for underactive bladder will now follow:~~

Treatments available for underactive bladder
↑

> With this heading the preliminary sentence is made redundant.

~~The results are provided next~~

Results

Here is another example where a phrase is not adding any new information.

The participants were allowed to withdraw at any point during the session ~~*if they decided they did not want to continue participating in the study*~~.

The same applies to tables. Rather than introducing the table and then repeating this in the title, summarise the key point and let the actual table title and graphics do the rest.

The following table (2.3) shows the bacterial fermentation products formed from different carbohydrates.   ✗

It seems that not all FC substrates produce an equal amount of SCFA (Table 2.3)   ✓

Table 2.3: Bacterial fermentation products formed from different carbohydrates

Move some data to tables

When writing out extensive results ask yourself whether they would be clearer to the reader and better served in a table. In this example the reader may eventually work out what the results mean or find a significant computational time, but analysis could be carried out quicker if the data were presented in a table.

During the third task, the mean computational times per frame during the global optimisation for models A, A2, B3, C, and D are 89 ± 38 ms/fr, 75 ± 28 ms/fr, 103 ± 34 ms/fr, 87 ± 31 ms/fr, and 86 ± 39 ms/fr, respectively. For the fourth task, the mean computational times per frame for models A, A2, B3, C, and D are 86 ± 35 ms/fr, 78 ± 38 ms/fr, 93 ± 33 ms/fr, 92 ± 46 ms/fr, and 80 ± 37 ms/fr, respectively.

But avoid these redundant terms in table captions.

~~The~~ yellow ~~colour~~ shows no change; orange ~~in colour~~ represents the results on day 10.

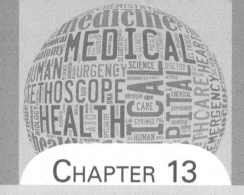

CHAPTER 13

Complaint M: Spelling and punctuation

> Signs:
> → Misspelling terms
> → Using the wrong punctuation

Treatment

Spelling errors in a paper can result from confusing two terms, using the wrong style or simply not taking care when typing. The following lists cover all three areas. Unlike some areas of English grammar that depend on understanding concepts, resolving spelling issues is simply about concentration and awareness.

Be aware of the most commonly misspelled words

The terms used in medicine and surgery are drawn from many sources and tend to either contain unusual letter combinations or sound and look like more mainstream terms. Familiarise yourself with the list and make sure you don't get caught out.

✗	✓	✗	✓
a posterior	**a posteriori**	irradation	**irradiation**
absess	**abscess**	lacunea	**lacunae**
ajuvant	**adjuvant**	linage	**lineage**
alelle	**allele**	lumber	**lumbar**
anurism	**aneurysm**	osteogensis	**osteogenesis**
arrythmia	**arrhythmia**	preforated	**perforated**
arteriol	**arteriole**	periostem	**periosteum**
asess	**assess**	phlem	**phlegm**
capilliary	**capillary**	practioner	**practitioner**
cocomintant	**concomitant**	preperation	**preparation**
coltured	**cultured**	prodome	**prodrome**
debridment	**debridement**	progeniter	**progenitor**
demelination	**demyelination**	referal	**referral**
doner	**donor**	resusitation	**resuscitation**
doze	**dose** (see a–z)	rythum	**rhythm**
emollent	**emollient**	saiety	**satiety**
enviroment	**environment**	scaring	**scarring**
fatale	**fatal**	seperate	**separate**
fluoresent	**fluorescent**	strenous	**strenuous**
-gensis	**genesis**	supresses	**suppresses**
illic	**iliac**	sympton	**symptom**
in vitrio	**in vitro**	theraputic	**therapeutic**
intermitant	**intermittent**	tinitus	**tinnitus**
interstital	**interstitial**	venus	**venous**
intervenous	**intravenous**	vunerable	**vulnerable**

Some misspelled terms result from confusion with other words. Note their forms and definitions.

cite/site (to refer to, to quote/a position or location)

form/from (shape, to construct/a starting point or source)

incubation/intubation (maintenance of conditions to favour growth and development/insertion of a tube into the body)

log/lag (logarithmic growth/population remains constant)

prescribe/proscribe (to order the use of/to prohibit or ban)

proceed/precede (to carry on or continue/to come before)

prostate/prostrate (a gland in male mammals/lying face down, to lay flat)

ratio/ration (relation between quantities/a fixed amount)

relive/relieve (to experience again/to ease, to bring relief)

root/route (an essential part, an anchor/a way or path)

sac/sack (a bag-like structure in an animal/a large bag)

sever/severe (to separate, to break/extreme, critical)

serous/serious (relating to serum/unfavourable, grave)

stationary/stationery (fixed, standing still/writing materials)

vesical/vesicle (relating to a vesica or bladder/a sac or cyst)

waist/waste (the middle section/unused, to squander)

weighed/weighted (measure the weight of/adjusted or adapted to a certain value)

wheel/wheal (a circular frame/an itching or burning swelling)

Pairs of terms that require a more thorough examination can be found in the a–z section.

Know the differences between AE and BE

It is important to know in advance whether British English or American English is required. The main differences in spelling are captured in this list of common medical terms:

AE	BE	AE	BE
acclimation	*acclimatisation*	etiology	*aetiology*
analyze	*analyse*	fecal	*faecal*
anemia	*anaemia*	fetal	*foetal*
anesthetic	*anaesthetic*	gonorrhea	*gonorrhoea*
behavior	*behaviour*	hemoglobin	*haemoglobin*
catalyze	*catalyse*	hemorrhage	*haemorrhage*
categorize*	*categorise*	labor	*labour*
cesarean	*caesarian*	maneuver	*manoeuvre*
characterize	*characterise*	meter	*metre*
celiac	*coeliac*	odor	*odour*
dialyzer	*dialyser*	paralyze	*paralyse*
diarrhea	*diarrhoea*	pediatrics	*paediatrics*
distill	*distil*	recognize	*recognise*
edema	*oedema*	sulfur	*sulphur*
enroll	*enrol*	tumor	*tumour*
esophagus	*oesophagus*	vapor	*vapour*
estrogen	*oestrogen*		

Master apostrophe use

The apostrophe is used to indicate both possession and contraction. It is used to show that something belongs to someone or something or to a group. Note that the apostrophe comes before the 's' for these singular nouns and after the 's' for the plural nouns.

author　　*author's*　　*authors'*

country　　*country's*　　*countries'*

patient　　*patient's*　　*patients'*

*The **authors'** biographies are presented at the end of the paper.* (plural: more than one author)

*The **author's** biography is presented at the end of the paper.* (singular: one author)

---

* The Oxford English Dictionary recommends "-ize" endings also as standard.

INTERVENTION   **it's**

Of course the classic possessive error is its/it's

its – *The most important feature is ~~it's~~ (**its**) lack of side effects.*
it's = (it is)

---

*The ~~participants'~~ (**participants**) were then asked to...*

There appears to be an urge to use the possessive
apostrophe with almost every plural noun. In the
example above there is no possession taking place
so no apostrophe is required.

Some writers use the possessive apostrophe for inanimate objects,
while others argue the of-phrase is the only acceptable form. A compound form with a generic meaning and without an apostrophe or
an of-phrase is also starting to gain favour. But the specific or generic
nature of the sentence should determine which option to take.

We will also look at the device's suitability.

We will also look at the suitability of the device.

We will also look at device suitability.

When the sentence is not generic and a specific entity is being referred
to, the first two options are available.

*The patient's data should have been entered into the system that
stores patient data.*

Here a specific patient is being referred
to so the apostrophe form is appropriate.

Now we have the more general reference
and the generic third form is appropriate.

Contractions are discouraged in academic writing.

*We ~~don't~~ (**do not**) test for this until stage five is complete.*

And apostrophes are not required for abbreviations or dates.

~~BMSC's~~ **BMSCs** ~~1990's~~ **1990s**

The use of apostrophes for terms that contain a person's name is common; however, the process is fairly random and there are many diseases, treatments and parts of the body named after people that do not contain an apostrophe. As always, check the form of a specific term from a reliable source. The following partial list will demonstrate the point:

With an apostrophe	*Without an apostrophe*
Addison's disease	Apgar score
Auerbach's plexus	Arnold–Chiari malformation
Babinski's reflex/Babinski reflex	Barr body
Baker's cyst	Bence Jones protein
Bankart's operation	Braxton Hicks contractions
Barlow's disease	Brown-Séquard syndrome
Bartholin's glands	Budd–Chiari syndrome
Basedow's disease	Caldwell–Luc operation…

Distinguish the dashes

-   hyphen   – en dash   — em dash

Hyphens are the smallest of the three horizontal lines. They connect words and word fragments but should be adopted sparingly.

They are used for the following:

In compounds that are modifying a noun and coming before the noun (see also Complaint F)

*We noted an increased intake of **energy-dense** foods.*

but not after the noun

*The different stages of the condition have been **well defined** (5).*

or if the modifier is complex

For this we use the **waist-to-hip** *ratio.*

> If the words include an adverb ending in –ly, a comparative/superlative or they are a pair of words not directly connected to the final noun, do not use a hyphen.
>
> *This is a* **newly installed machine** *that can detect...*
>
> *Next we discuss the small,* **positive steps that can be taken**....

or if the prefix part of the word ends in a vowel and the next part begins with the same vowel

The issue relates to whether it will then **re-emerge** *in a different area...*

> There are a couple of exceptions to this:
>
> *cooperate/cooperation*   *coordinate/coordination*

or for double names

It was generated from the plasma concentration profiles using the **Wagner-Nelson** *method.*

> **ASSESSMENT**   **The suspended hyphen**
>
> When two or more hyphenated terms end the same way, the first phrase can be suspended at the hyphen. The noun(s)/adjective(s) are then attached only to the final term of the set.
>
> **This is true for both the 2w- and 4w-disuse groups.*

– en dash

The en dash is the length of a standard 'n' and is used mainly for notation to represent ranges and to split up names and opposites.

2001–2007   pp. 110–118   –22°C   true–false test

– em dash

The em dash is slightly longer than the hyphen and the en dash and has two functions. It is used at the end of a sentence for a final thought or a restatement of a previous thought. It is especially useful in long sentences when a set of commas has already been used. Only one dash is used for this task.

The data is available to all practitioners, especially data related to the outcomes of relevant trials, but training is required on effective search techniques—as observed in our study.

It can also be used in pairs instead of commas or parentheses to add emphasis and to clarify, or if the phrase interrupts the previous one. Parentheses should be used for interruption if the phrase carries little importance.

If the infant has reached a suitable weight—usually around 5 kg—then dialysis would also be available.

Do not use two en dashes or hyphens side by side for an em dash.   --✗

Be conscious of the comma

Punctuation is used to organise writing, enhance readability and promote understanding. Too much punctuation or too little will make for an unpleasant reading experience; the wrong punctuation will obscure and even completely change the meaning of a sentence. The position of the comma changes the meaning of these sentences:

Six healthy subjects were given rectal infusions containing acetate (90 mmol) plus propionate (30 mmol), acetate (180 mmol) plus propionate (60 mmol), or saline.

> Without the final comma the infusions change completely.
> Without the comma saline is administered with acetate and with the comma the saline is administered alone.

Approximately 70% of the acetate production, which is exogenous acetate formed by colonic bacterial fermentation, is taken up by the liver.

> Without the first comma the 70% is exogenous acetate and with the comma the exogenous acetate is merely further information about the acetate.

Commas should not be used to split up sentences that are independent and represent two different thoughts—that is the role of full stops. Here a full stop should begin the sentence 'The results showed…'

To assess the clinical relevance of___ we analysed the relevant data, the results showed that....

Limit the capitals

Capital letters are always overused. Only names of places, companies, organisations and people should be given capitals; this usually includes people who have given their name to diseases, signs, methods, etc.

Dr Ravi Benson   Indonesia

the Red Cross   Stargardt disease

AstraZeneca   Michael

Remember to use capital letters for every author.

This was noted by Morgan and ~~jones~~ *(Jones).*

In taxonomy, the genus is always capitalised and the species lower case.

Rattus norvegicus

Terms that should have capital letters but that are commonly written without include

✗	✓
abo system	**ABO** system
angle/bundle of his	angle/bundle of **His**
asian flu	**Asian** flu
circle of willis	circle of **Willis**
crypts of lieberkühn	crypts of **Lieberkühn**
d-dimer assay	**D**-dimer assay
data protection act	**Data Protection Act**
organ of corti	organ of **Corti**
q wave	**Q** wave
rem sleep	**REM** sleep
rh negative/positive	**Rh** negative/positive
t cell	**T** cell
the Nhs	the **NHS**
a uti	a **UTI**
vitamin a,b	vitamin **A, B**...

The inaccurate and seemingly arbitrary use of capital letters by some writers is ably reflected in the following passage. NONE of the terms in bold require a capital letter.

> Although **Tinnitus** is associated with hearing loss, other medical factors must be considered as possible causes. These factors include conditions such as **Vascular** disease, diabetes, **Hypertension**, autoimmune disorders and degenerative neural disorder with or without **Concomitant Hearing Loss**. In addition, these medical conditions usually are accompanied by using medication that may lead to **Tinnitus** emergence or exacerbation. Typically, **Subjective Tinnitus** can be perceived as **Ringing**, buzzing, hissing, whistling or humming.

Place the parentheses

Parentheses are used in the main text to enclose a non-restrictive clause that adds information but has no real bearing on, or importance to, the sentence as a whole.

The relative acute angle between the longitudinal axes (also known as the carrying angle) is taken into account...

Parentheses are also employed for the manufacturer's details when describing the equipment used.

This was placed in a diamond-coated grinding system (EXAKT Apparatebau GmbH & Co, Norderstedt, Germany; EX AKT Medical Instruments, Oklahoma City, OK).

CASE REPORT: COLON TREATMENT

Colons should not be used to introduce items mid-sentence.

The treatment effect was rated: excellent/good or fair/poor. ✗

They can introduce lists if the sentence is a complete one and are often used after the terms following/as follows.

Exclusion criteria were as follows:

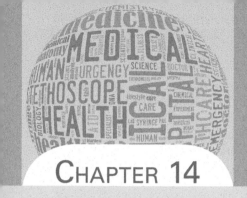

CHAPTER 14

Complaint N: Titles

> Signs:
> → Using a title that is irrelevant and unhelpful

Treatment

This section presents the rules and regulations for producing a title for your work. As the first piece of text the reader sees, titles need to be relevant (reliable), effective (persuasive) and appropriately edited (professional). But for the reader to see it in today's world of accessing content electronically, it also needs to feature both conventional terms and key words.

Compare the following*:

A Study using a prospective Randomized comparing of oral Sodium posphate, and also polyethylene glycol lavage for the preperation of a Colonoscopy

Prospective Randomized Comparison of Oral Sodium Phosphate and Polyethylene Glycol Lavage for Colonoscopy Preparation

---

* Original titles modified for illustrative purposes.

Select a title that suits your paper

The main title should inform the reader of the nature of the work as succinctly as possible. Only key terms should be used and adjectives and introductory statements avoided, unless fundamental to the paper. Remember that the abstract will provide the necessary detail for the reader to fully assess the work.

Let's evaluate the two titles provided earlier:

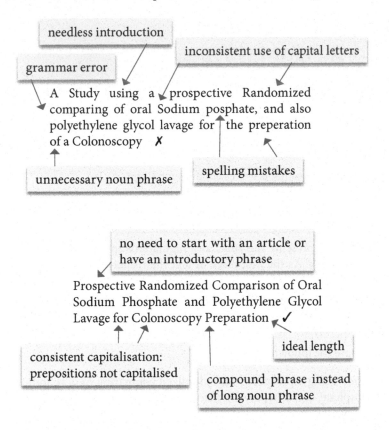

The title content will depend on the nature of the paper. It is useful to include the type of study in the title or subtitle.

Randomised Single-blind Trial of...   *Clinical Study of the...*

Bowel Obstruction: a Case Report...

For review papers or descriptive works that focus on a particular structure, the subject often appears at the start followed by a colon or dash and a subtitle.

Streptococcus Pneumoniae – Prevalence and Risk Factors...

The title should contain information about how the topic is being approached. Is it a general analysis? Are the effects or implications of something being looked at? Is something being identified? Are guidelines being presented? Has the method or device been explicitly stated?

Identification and Characterisation of a Novel Family of Pneumococcal Proteins that are Protective against Sepsis

Guidelines for Preoperative Fasting and Use of Pharmacologic Agents to Reduce the Risk of Pulmonary Aspiration

Some general or mainstream journals prefer more informal, sometimes even satirical, titles. Check past issues for the type of headings that are appropriate and welcomed.

INTERVENTION   **proclaiming**

Avoid titles that make an assertion or claim and that announce the key finding. Try to rephrase or pose a question.

Polyphenols have a direct effect on the balance of the major groups of gut microbiota   ✗

Effect of polyphenols on the balance of the major groups of gut microbiota   ✓

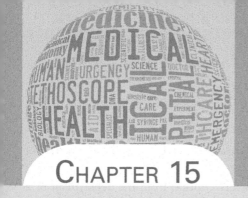

CHAPTER 15

Complaint O: References

> Signs:
> → Failing to cite correctly in the main text
> → Creating an unsatisfactory reference list

Treatment

To ensure that the references are in the correct format, the website of the relevant journal or the school department should be consulted. Students who search for a general guide to the Vancouver style or AMA/BMJ style may receive conflicting information. Issues like spacing, colons, italics for titles and date/month placement are common inconsistencies in guidelines found on the Internet.

For instance, one site states that three authors should be written out before et al (or 'others') is inserted, but then offers up this example: Morgan S, *et al.*

Another site instructs the author to italicise journal titles and then proceeds to give an example without the title in italics.

Another presents a reference guide for medical students and then uses examples from engineering and geology.

It was therefore considered more helpful to demonstrate the areas on which to concentrate and the signs to look out for than provide a strict set of examples that may not be relevant for the particular institute or journal receiving your work.

So, to make sure your references are in the correct format take the following three steps:

- Contact the department or relevant journal to obtain an example of the correct format.
- Examine a recent essay or dissertation from the department or a published article from the journal to confirm the format.
- Compile the reference list and then ask a trusted colleague to check it for you.

Utilise the number system

Most medical institutes and journals use the number system to cite work in the main text; however, there are variations with formatting so you should check with the journal or school you are submitting to. The three types of in-text number citation are round brackets outside the punctuation, square brackets inside the punctuation and superscript.

These may degrade RNA molecules at different rates and by different mechanisms.(7–9)

Others have developed multiplex assays composed of a number of body fluid-specific transcripts [5, 8, 13, 15].

A previous study[12] has shown that degradation is related to…

As each work is mentioned in the text it is given a number. If the same work is mentioned again it retains its original number. For more than one work the style is as follows:

…used a different technique. (7, 8, 9)   ✗

…used a different technique. (7–9)   ✓

…used a different technique. (7–9) (12, 14, 15, 16)   ✗

…used a different technique. (7–9, 12, 14–16)   ✓

When using the number system keep the brackets free of names or other information.

It is important to consider the unique characteristics of the D gene when performing a compatibility test (7 ~~Morgan~~).

ASSESSMENT   **name–year referencing**

Some biological science journals and departments use the Harvard system or the name–year method. In-text:

Cui (2009) recruited healthy obese Japanese volunteers and randomised them...

If the source is being directly referred to in the text then only put brackets around the date.

(Zhao & Stephens 1998) investigated the similarities...   ✗

Zhao & Stephens (1998) investigated the similarities...   ✓

A common error is

A study ~~of~~ (by) Morgan (1998) tested the effectiveness of...

The references are then created alphabetically.

Cui, H, (2009)...

Douglas, J, (2001)...

Evans, TM, (1987)...

Know what to look for

Attention should be focused on these areas.

Names –

Should the initials come before or after the surnames? Should there be spaces, dots and/or commas between the names and initials?

When should *et al.* be used if at all?

Month/Year –

Should the year be after the authors or at the end?

> Make sure the year has not been written twice in the reference

Should there be brackets around the year?
Should the month be included? Where should it go?

Italics –

Should the titles of books and journals be in italics and/or have initial capital letters?
Should the volume and/or page numbers be in italics?

Numbers and spacing –

Should 'vol' or 'volume' be written for journals?
Should there be spaces between the number and page numbers?
Should there be spaces between the author's initials?

Publisher –

Should the location come before or after the publisher?
Should the location be abbreviated?

Journal titles are abbreviated for most reference styles in medicine.

> *Shantry, K. Developments in wound care.* **Am J Nurs**. 2006
> Aug 9;311(5):230–237 ↑
>
> American Journal of Nursing

Here are a select few with their associated errors:

FULL TERM	ABBREVIATION	ERROR
Abstracts	**Abstr**	~~Abs~~
Adolescent	**Adolesc**	~~Adol~~
Anatomic/Anatomy	**Anat**	~~Anatom~~
Annals	**Ann**	~~Annal~~
Annual	**Annu**	~~Ann~~
Biology/Biological	**Biol**	~~Bio~~
British	**Br**	~~Brit~~
Carbohydrate	**Carbohydr**	~~Carb~~
Diagnosis/Diagnostics	**Diagn**	~~Diag~~
Disorder(s)	**Disord**	~~Dis~~
Emergency	**Emerg**	~~Emerge~~
European	**Eur**	~~Europe~~
Infection/Infectious	**Infect**	~~Inf~~
Institute	**Inst**	~~Ins~~
Joint	**Jt**	~~Join~~
Letters	**Lett**	~~Letts~~
Materials	**Mater**	~~Mat~~
Maternal	**Matern**	~~Mat~~
Oncology	**Oncol**	~~Onc~~
Organic	**Org**	~~Organ~~
Organization	**Organ**	~~Org~~
Paediatrica/Paediatric	**Paediatr**	~~Paed~~

(*Continued*)

FULL TERM	ABBREVIATION	ERROR
Proceedings	**Proc**	~~Pro~~
Rehabilitation	**Rehabil**	~~Rehab~~
Transfusion	**Transfus**	~~Trans~~

Eliminate agreement and grammar errors

Make sure that the numbers used in the text match with those in the reference list.

A 12 day cross-over trial was also conducted by Whelan (6).

6. Zung, W.W., *From art to science. The diagnosis and treatment of depression...*

Make sure that a reference has not been repeated. If it has then the numbers will obviously need reallocating.

7. Brown, R.F., et al. Relationship between stress and relapse in multiple sclerosis. *Mult Scler*, 2006. **12**(4): p. 465–75.
8. Brown, R.F., et al. Relationship between stress and relapse in multiple sclerosis. *Mult Scler*, 2006. **12**(4): p. 465–75.

Make sure you have captured all the inconsistencies among entries, no matter how minor.

Aaron DM, Charles J, Regan M. Developments in dementia. Arch Neurol. 2001 Jan;54(1):96–109.

Allen P.K., W. Cho. Six Frameworks for Dementia Programs. *Arch Neurol.* (2003) Mar;68 2,134—148.

Note the differences in the second entry

second author name and initial reversed	capitals for words in title
period between initials	no brackets around issue number
italics for journal title	colon replaced with comma
brackets around year	em dash for page range

Make sure that a reference in the list has been referred to in the text. Naturally this will have an impact on the number order if the list was compiled before the work had been completed. A 'works consulted' section could be added depending on the specific guidelines.

– further errors

The treatment plans devised by John Mitchell-Matthews (4) have long been admired for their...

---

4. ~~Matthews JM~~. Treatment of...

4. ~~Matthews J Mitchell~~. Treatment of...

4. ~~Matthews-Mitchell J~~. Treatment of...

*4. **Mitchell-Matthews J**. Treatment of...*

*Trang L. Treatment of cortical contusion injury. Brain Res. ~~Forthcoming~~ (**Forthcoming**) 2016.*

*~~Dissertation:~~ Ball NL. New approaches in adolescent care [**dissertation**]. Falmouth (UK). University of ____; 2010*

*Abuka L. The health care response to the Ebola outbreak... Available ~~at~~ (**from**): http://www.nun.org/files/ebola/14.*

...is a primary concern (Dupon et al., 2013, Dupon et al., 2014). ✗

...is a primary concern (Dupon et al., 2013; 2014). ✓

A–Z list of errors

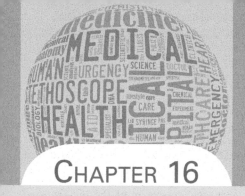

CHAPTER 16

A–Z list of errors

absent/absence

absent – adjective

absence – noun

The noun does have a countable form but is usually uncountable. Confusing the noun with the adjective is common.

*They were ~~absence~~ (**absent**) from the trial.*

*The ~~absent~~ (**absence**) of these three participants was noted.*

active/activate

active adjective – engaged in action; physically energetic

activate verb – to make active or cause to function

*This toxin ~~actives~~ (**activates**) guanylate cyclase and this can lead to diarrhoea.*

The verb is also mistakenly used instead of the plural noun 'activities'.

*Fatigue was apparent even when performing routine ~~activates~~ (**activities**).*

accurate/accuracy

accurate – adjective
accuracy – noun

*The program requires the collection of ~~accuracy~~ (**accurate**) intake data.*

Selecting the adjective instead of the noun is a very common error.

*We would also question the ~~accurate~~ (**accuracy**) of the self-reported questionnaire.*

adduction/abduction

Keep an eye on these two opposites. One is a limb moving away from the body and the other is towards.

adduction – drawing or moving a limb towards the middle of the body
abduction – moving a limb away from the middle of the body

*This can be tested by **abduction** of the arm.*

*Morgan and colleagues carried out a study on knee **adduction**...*

adjust/adjustment

Sometimes the simple present third person singular (it adjusts, he/she adjusts) is mistakenly used instead of the associated plural noun. Adjust/adjustment is a good example of this type of error.

adjust – verb

adjustment – noun

*The necessary ~~adjusts~~ (**adjustments**) have been made to the method.*

adopt/adapt

adopt – to select, choose or take as one's own; to follow

adapt – to adjust or modify to suit a new purpose; to adjust to different conditions

If you adopt something (such as a routine, model, technique or programme) you select it or follow it without changing it. If you adapt it you make changes to it to suit your own needs.

*Although elderly participants tried to ~~adapt~~ (**adopt**) this strategy to cope initially, they soon…*

*It is also important they ~~adopt~~ (**adapt**) to their changing health needs.*

*The first model and the secondary stages were **adapted** from Morgan (2009; 2011).*

adverse/averse

adverse – unfavourable or opposite

averse – having a strong feeling of opposition

Both are adjectives but can be distinguished. 'adverse' usually refers to conditions or actions that are negative or unfavourable. 'averse' means to be opposed to something or to be reluctant to do something and describes a person's attitudes or feelings. Some errors involve simply forgetting to add the 'd' rather than any real mix up in meaning.

*This has been known to bring about ~~averse~~ (**adverse**) effects.*

Aversion and averse are usually followed by 'to'

*Patients often complain of an aversion ~~about~~ (**to**) fatty foods.*

advice/advise

advice – noun

advise – verb

'advice' is an uncountable noun and therefore does not have a plural form (~~advices~~). The verb form is required in all of these sentences:

*It is still too early to ~~advice~~ (**advise**) the use of polyphenols as a strategy here.*

*Patients should be ~~adviced~~ (**advised**) to reduce their alcohol and salt intake.*

*This study ~~advices~~ (**advises**) an anti-human globulin along with the use of...*

When seeking advice the preposition choice will depend on the situation:

They should seek the advice of (someone)

They should seek advice from (someone)

They should seek advice on (a matter, an illness/condition)

afferent/efferent

afferent – bearing inward or toward an organ or part of the body

efferent – conducting outward or away from an organ or part of the body

Here is another pair of opposites. a- is inward and e- is outward.

Afferent signals may include these nerves or hormones.

Next we investigate the efferent function in participants with normal hearing.

agree/accept

There is overlap here but 'agree' is often used with 'to' or 'with' and 'accept' is usually followed by a noun.

accept   agreed to   agreed with

*In the end, sixteen patients ~~accepted~~ (**agreed**) to participate.*

*It is important to **accept** these age-related changes...*

analysis/analyse

analyse – verb

analysis – noun (plural: analyses)

*...and then confirm the tissue type of the ~~analysis~~ (**analysed**) sample*

*This will follow a critical ~~analyse~~ (**analysis**) of the issue.*

Remember to use the plural form of the noun as it is often overlooked. It has the same form as the verb in the third person singular.

*Many ~~analysis~~ (**analyses**) have failed to consider the underlying issues.*

The preposition 'of' is used after the noun.

*There will also be an ~~analysis about~~ (**analysis of**) evolving treatments.*

anamnesis

This means the case history of a patient, particularly their background, experiences and recollections in order to effectively analyse their condition. If used in an essay or paper, an explanation of the term would be of help to the reader.

anomaly/anomalous

anomaly   noun – something that is unusual or unexpected

anomalous   adjective – not expected; unusual or uncertain

Often the adjective form and the plural noun are mixed.

*These may explain the ~~anomalous~~ (**anomalies**) in the results of the ABO blood grouping.*

*The cardiovascular ~~anomalous~~ (**anomalies**) include coarctation of the aorta.*

Here is a mistake with the singular form:

*This is considered a slightly more common congenital ~~anomalous~~ (**anomaly**).*

Anomalous is perhaps most often seen in the term 'anomalous pulmonary venous connection'.

basic/basis

basic adjective – essential; underlying

basis noun – the main principle, the foundation

*The models may be used on an application-specific ~~basic~~ (**basis**).*

*This is a ~~basis~~ (**basic**) principle of this system.*

Also 'base' is required when referring to the lower or lowest part of something.

*This was noted at the ~~basis~~ (**base**) of the left lung.*

benefit/beneficial

Benefit can be a noun or a verb.

*This **benefits** not only the caregivers but also the immediate family.*

*The recommended frequency is five times a week to maximise the **benefit**.*

Beneficial is the adjective form.

*These anthocyanins are associated with ~~benefit~~ (**beneficial**) health effects.*

Benefit is often found with 'from'

*Those experiencing gastrointestinal symptoms may well **benefit from** gluten withdrawal.*

There is also a fixed phrase 'of benefit'.

*Altering the seat position may be ~~of a benefit~~ (**of benefit**).*

blockage

Although it can be a noun, 'block' is more often utilised as a verb with 'blockage' the associated noun. The noun can be countable or uncountable as seen in these examples.

*This difficulty is the result of partial or complete ~~block~~ (**blockage**).*

*Many experienced incomplete evacuation and a ~~block~~ (**blockage**) in the anus.*

breakdown

breakdown – noun
break down – phrasal verb

Some compounds can be separated to become phrasal verbs (see Chapter 1). **This is the case with 'breakdown', where the noun is one word and the verb two.**

*This is a result of increased ~~break down~~ (**breakdown**) of red blood cells.*

*Several enzymes are believed to ~~breakdown~~ (**break down**) this tissue.*

breath/breathe

breath – noun
breathe – verb

Think about whether you need the verb or the noun here because it is a common mistake.

*The next step is the glucose hydrogen ~~breathe~~ (**breath**) tests.*

*The participants were instructed to ~~breath~~ (**breathe**) normally...*

bypass

This is always one word and cannot be turned into a phrasal verb. Also keep an eye on the spelling.

*These symptoms are markedly improved after gastric ~~by pass~~ (**bypass**).*

*Two other bariatric procedures are gastric ~~bipass~~ (**bypass**) and sleeve gastrectomy.*

called

Do not add 'as' when you are stating what something is called.

Others disagree that patients should be called ~~as~~ clients.

The same applies to 'named' and 'termed'.

This fatigue inventory contains three factors (named ~~as~~ physical, mental and spiritual).

Perhaps the confusion stems from the term 'known as'.

cardiac/cardial

Both adjectives relate to the heart. It is best to check reliable sources for the accepted adjective used in a particular term. A few are listed here:

cardiac arrest	myocardial infarction
cardiac cycle	cardial glands
cardiac failure	cardial notch
cardiac valve	cardial orifice

carry out

Opt for 'carry out' instead of forms of the verb 'to do' when referring to research or trials.

*Three in vitro fermentation experiments were ~~done~~ (**carried out**) to validate...*

*It is not possible to ~~do~~ (**carry out**) such a study with humans because of ethical considerations.*

causal/casual

'casual', which means relaxed or unconcerned, is often confused with 'causal', which refers to a cause.

*We will aim to establish a ~~casual~~ (**causal**) relationship between the variables.*

The noun 'causality' is the relationship between cause and effect.

cause/course

cause   noun – something that produces an effect

            verb – to bring about; to be the reason for

course   noun – the path or route taken; a program of education or medication

If there is genuine confusion about which is which, just think of a racecourse or a golf course as a route. In medicine 'course' often refers to the path that a disease or condition takes over time.

*Their study looked at the prevalence and clinical **course** of functional dyspepsia.*

*These genetic alterations are a major ~~course~~ (**cause**) of cancer initiation.*

A third term that has a similar sound is 'coarse', an adjective describing something made up of large particles or rough material.

*Food with **coarse** particles is less readily digested than the finer particles found in many…*

cease/seize

cease – to discontinue; to stop; to come to an end

seize – to take hold; to take possession or control

The verbs are often confused.

*ADH production will then ~~seize~~ (**cease**), leading to rapid excretion from the kidneys.*

The derived noun 'seizure' is also likely to occur in medical papers. 'Cessation' is the noun form of 'cease'.

*We will now look at the consequences of growth hormone **cessation**…*

cleansing/cleaning

Both are used to describe the removal of dirt and unwanted substances. Cleanse has a more thorough and technical connotation than clean as illustrated in the procedure of 'colonic cleansing'.

The ~~cleaning~~ *(**cleansing**) rate for the colon was the second measure we used.*

cofounding/confounding

cofounding – establishing something with another person or others

confounding – a third variable interfering with other variables to distort an association being studied (statistics)

Confounding and its associated forms are usually what the writer is seeking.

This analysis was used to calculate the ratios and correct for potential ~~cofounders~~ *(**confounders**) like gender and age.*

colic/colicky

colic – noun

colicky – adjective

Spelling is an issue here along with forgetting to use the quirky adjective when necessary.

The pain ranged from mild to severe with spontaneous ~~colic~~ *(**colicky**) spasms.*

This gastrointestinal disorder has also been suggested as a cause of ~~colick~~ *(**colic**).*

complain/complaint

complain – verb

complaint – noun

We complain about something and a complaint can be made to somebody.

*Her main ~~complain~~ (**complaint**) was with the clinic and the way it handled her initial...*

In this next example, complaint can be used if it was a particular instance of discontent that occurred rather than a general criticism.

*They also heard the staff ~~complaint~~ (**complain**) about the conditions on the ward.*

Some consider it inappropriate to use the verb to refer to a patient describing symptoms or an ailment because it gives the impression that the patient is moaning; was suffering from, reported, described and was experiencing are preferred.

Patient B ~~complained about~~ a tingling sensation down one side of their body.

*Patient B **reported** a tingling sensation down one side of their body.*

compliment/complement

complement   noun – something that adds to or completes something else

compliment   noun – an expression of praise

Both have verb forms identical to the noun: 'to complement' and 'to compliment'.

*The next section discusses how these two procedures actually ~~compliment~~ (**complement**) each other.*

*They are not used to receiving ~~complements~~ (**compliments**) about their smile.*

The therapy will require the first of the two nouns.

Complementary therapies attempt to treat the whole person rather than one specific aspect...

concern

verb – to relate to

*This section **concerns** the fermentation models of the colon.*

verb – to trouble or worry

*They were especially **concerned** about the potential side effects.*

The following situations require 'consider' not 'concern':

*Morgan and colleagues ~~concern~~ (**consider**) such a treatment in (11) and (12).*

*Both physical and mental aspects were ~~concerned~~ (**considered**) when analysing this.*

'concern' is also a countable noun.

*In the focus group there were **concerns** about the length of the trial.*

concurrent/current

concurrent – occurring at the same time, simultaneous

current – most recent; present

Only use concurrent when two or more things are being described.

*Their ~~concurrent~~ (**current**) condition is stable and they will likely be monitored for...*

*They documented **concurrent** drug therapy for tuberculosis and HIV infection.*

congenital

Spelling is the issue here. Note these two errors.

*This type of anaemia may be ~~cogenital~~ (**congenital**) or acquired.*

*~~Congential~~ (**Congenital**) disorders are covered in the next section.*

conscious/conscience

conscious – aware of oneself; awake

conscience – an inner sense of what is right and wrong

These two look similar and also sound similar as the ending of the latter is shortened when pronounced. The former is the medical term, the latter the moral one.

*It is characterised by increasing confusion and a loss of ~~conscienceness~~ (**consciousness**).*

consequently/subsequently

consequently – as a result

subsequently – next, following

There is some overlap here, but strictly speaking 'consequently' is when the following part is 'because of' the previous part.

*Observational studies typically include a broader population and are less costly. ~~Subsequently~~ (**Consequently**), they are chosen over...*

Use subsequently simply to show something happened afterwards. Often there is cause involved as well but the link is not necessarily as important.

*The patients arrived and were **subsequently** shown to the main reception.*

*As a ~~subsequence~~ (**consequence**) of this, we lengthened the trial to four weeks.*

'subsequence' is restricted to mathematics.

*Next, count the number of ways R is obtained **as a subsequence** of P.*

consult/consultation

consult – verb

consultation – noun

'Consult' is increasingly being used as a noun but this is informal use and 'consultation' is preferred in academic writing.

*They are likely to seek a **consultation** with this increase in the number of episodes.*

consume/consumption

consume – verb

consumption – noun

This is typical verb/noun confusion. The second sentence could be rewritten as 'consuming starch' but the noun works better for reporting the association.

*The ~~consume~~ (**consumption**) of 10 g/day of total dietary fibre was…*

*There was a weak association between starch ~~consuming~~ (**consumption**) and large bowel cancer incidence…*

contrary/contrast

~~In the contrary~~   Use **On the contrary**

~~In the contrast~~   Use **In contrast**

~~In contrary to~~   Use **Contrary to**

On the contrary, the first intervention failed to achieve a single reduction.

In contrast, our data have been collected over a much shorter period.

Contrary to the findings in (32) we found no instances at all.

There is little general difference between the phrases, but 'in contrast' is normally used as a mere comparison whereas the other two ('on the contrary'/ 'contrary to') are used to clearly state the opposite and show disagreement.

'On the contrary' can only be used as a response to something just mentioned.

~~On the contrary~~ to the findings of Morgan…

*The findings are not disappointing as previous reports claim; **on the contrary**, they provide a number of interesting…*

Defect

The noun and adjective forms are linked.

defect   noun – a fault or imperfection
defective   adjective – faulty; imperfect

But the verb is unrelated and 'defected' is not used in medicine.

*The next step is to replace the ~~defected~~ (**defective**) equipment.*

Genes, chemical/biological processes and machines tend to be defective. Defects tend to refer to heart issues and the treatment of bones.

Selecting the correct form is the main issue.

*At week 5, the ~~defective~~ (**defect**) was completely covered with newly formed bone...*

deficient/deficiency

deficient – adjective
deficiency – noun

Again, this is either a simple mix up of word endings or a failure to recognise the situations in which the forms are required.

A person can be deficient in something and they can have a deficiency.

*Bone marrow is also affected as an individual becomes iron ~~deficiency~~ (**deficient**).*

*Growth hormone ~~deficient~~ (**deficiency**) is an endocrine condition impacting on...*

descriptive/description

description – noun
descriptive – adjective

Descriptive should not be employed as a noun.

*A thorough ~~descriptive~~ (**description**) would be required for the clinic to process...*

*The other type of information is **descriptive** and this provides...*

detect/detection

detect – verb

detection – noun

detectable – adjective

The verb and the noun are mixed up on occasion.

*Narrow band imaging enhancement could improve the ~~detect~~ (**detection**) of gastric anisakis.*

The adjective should not be overlooked as it is far better than 'able to be detected'.

*The pattern was **detectable** because of the size of our sample for this trial.*

develop/development

develop – verb

development – noun

The noun is a classic example of having both countable and uncountable uses, but first of all ensure the verb has not been mistakenly used.

*The rapid ~~develop~~ (**development**) of new symptoms or complications would be another reason.*

countable – *The rapid developments in both technology and...*

uncountable – *This area is in dire need of development.*

diagnosed as/with

These are similar but the following is common usage:

Use 'diagnosed as' when referring to the disease or condition.

This has been diagnosed as non-bullous impetigo.

'diagnosed with' is generally avoided when directly referring to the patient

*This is also true of patients ~~diagnosed with~~ (**with**) breast cancer.*

'diagnosed by' is used to refer to the way in which the condition can be investigated:

This is often diagnosed by MRI scanning.

diagnostic/diagnosis

diagnostic – adjective   diagnostics – noun

diagnosis – noun

*They addressed the clinical consequences, ~~diagnosis~~ (**diagnostic**) approach and the treatment options.*

*As this can be a difficult ~~diagnostic~~ (**diagnosis**), chest radiographs should be...*

The practice of diagnosis is known as diagnostics.

discontinue/leave

discontinue – to end something

leave – to give up or stop participating in something

A researcher discontinues a study whereas a participant leaves it.

*Three of the participants ~~discontinued~~ (**left**) the study on the second day.*

*At six months the study was **discontinued**, with all participants...*

distend/distention

distend   verb – to swell out or cause to expand

*Constipation can cause the bowel to ~~distention~~ (**distend**), putting pressure on the bladder.*

There is a noun form that can be spelled either distention or distension.

distribute/distribution

distribute – verb

distribution – noun

The verb is used for something spreading or dispersing and the noun is often employed as a statistical term.

*These participants were at the upper end of the normal ~~distribute~~ (**distribution**).*

*It is ingested and ~~distribution~~ (**distributed**) to the target tissue where it is then potentially stored.*

disuse

Models of 'disuse' are tested, not 'disused.' Do not use the adjective form to name the model.

Muscle girth changes also appear in other ~~disused~~ *(disuse) models...*

dominant/dominate

dominant – adjective

dominance – noun

dominate – verb

Those suffering from a disease in which fatigue was the ~~dominate~~ *(dominant) symptom were excluded.*

Also take care with these forms:

predominant – adjective   predominantly – adverb

predominate – verb   predominance – noun

The ~~predominate~~ *(predominant) cause is the reduction of coronary blood flow...*

This may lead to underestimating its bioavailability because it is not known what forms ~~predominant~~ *(predominate) in vivo.*

Nodular sclerosis was ruled out as this ~~predominant~~ *(predominantly) affects young adults.*

dose/dosage

A distinction can be made between the two. 'Dose' refers to the amount taken at one specific time and can be made plural. 'Dosage' refers to the duration or the frequency of the dose (twice a day for instance) and cannot be made plural.

Two separate ~~dosages~~ *(doses) produced fewer alterations than the single dose treatment...*

Keep an eye on the spelling.

Tolerance can occur with increased ~~dozes~~ *(doses).*

effect/affect

affect   verb – to have an influence on

effect   verb – to accomplish

*This may ~~effect~~ (**affect**) their quality of life.*

*This ~~affected~~ (**effected**) the change to more personalised care.*

More commonly, 'effect' is a noun meaning result or consequence.

*This had no ~~affect~~ (**effect**) on the outcome of either trial.*

Therefore, note the following:

*Patients in double-blinded clinical trials are warned of the adverse side ~~affects~~ (**effects**)...*

In psychology and psychiatry 'affect' can also mean an expressed emotional response.

eligible

eligible – qualified or suitable to be chosen

Do not confuse with illegible – not clear or decipherable.

*In the end there were 125 ~~illegible~~ (**eligible**) patients who became trial subjects.*

Before technology transformed administrative matters, a doctor's handwriting was said to always be illegible.

everyday

'everyday' is an adjective that means normal or typical.

'every day' means daily or each day.

*As a trainee I had to carry out this duty ~~everyday~~ (**every day**).*

*This is considered a basic need in ~~every day~~ (**everyday**) life.*

exceed/excess

exceed verb – to go beyond with regard to quantity, degree or rate

excess noun – an extreme degree; going beyond the limits

For some reason errors tend to occur when a modal is present.

*The major products of bacterial fermentation may ~~excess~~ (**exceed**) 150 mmol/L when...*

except for/apart from

'except for' excludes something or someone.

*The volumes revealed significant differences between the groups after the operation, **except for** groups 3 and 4 at 10 weeks.*

'apart from' can exclude OR include something or someone.

***Apart from** verbal difficulties, this particular group may express their negative emotions in a subtle manner.* (include)

*The liver helps to synthesise all circulating proteins **apart from** immunoglobulin.* (exclude)

The error is made when trying to use 'except for' to include something.

*~~Except for~~ (**Apart from**) influencing purchase behaviour, food advertising is also hypothesized to contribute to obesity through triggering...*

Be careful not to confuse 'for' and 'from' in these terms.

~~except from~~............ ~~apart for~~

expect/expectation

expect – verb

expectation – noun

The first error is simply noun/verb confusion. The second error could be rectified with the addition of a definite article (*higher than the expectation*), but the verb is a much better option.

*The ~~expect~~ (**expectation**) is that by the second year of training, the practitioner will...*

*The prevalence in adults was higher than ~~expectation~~ (**expected**) with an overall standardized...*

exploratory/explanatory

exploratory – exploring or examining (usually in relation to an operation)

explanatory – explaining and making clear

The related nouns are exploration and explanation. Do not be influenced by the verb 'explain' when forming the noun.

*A pathophysiological ~~explaination~~ (**explanation**) will also be provided.*

extend/extended

'extend' is a verb meaning to stretch out or increase.

*We **extended** this to five weeks...*

'extent' is a noun meaning the degree to which something extends.

*The **extent** of this distribution can be seen in the table below.*

The following error is commonly made:

*It is not really known to what ~~extend~~ (**extent**) environmental causes are responsible.*

The other noun form is spelled with an 's'.

*This can be tested by ~~extention~~ (**extension**) of the fingers.*

follows/following

The different forms and the typical errors are listed.

...will be explained in the ~~follow~~ parts: **following**

The advantages are described as ~~following~~: **follows**

The ~~followings~~ are some suggestions: **following**

to follow – verb to come after or next.

*An explanation of the pain-modulatory pathways will then **follow**.*

– verb to obey

*We **followed** the program developed in (9) and (15).*

following – noun that which comes immediately after

*This can be seen in the **following**:*

– adjective that which will now be described

*...as seen in the **following** table:*

as follows – adverb what is listed next

*The three possible treatments are **as follows**:*

frail/frailty

frail – adjective

frailty – noun

Note the application of the two forms:

With an ageing population, it is clear that many more people will become **frail** *during later life.*

With an ageing population, it is clear that many more people will experience **frailty** *during later life.*

A score above 5 indicates that the individual is ~~frailty~~ (**frail**).

harm/harmful

harm – noun or verb

harmful – adjective

As a noun 'harm' is uncountable so has no plural form.

The ~~harms~~ (**harm**) *of tobacco to non-smokers helped mobilize support for smoke-free legislation...*

We also reveal its ~~harm~~ (**harmful**) *effect and its negative economic consequences.*

imaging/imagining

imaging – creating visual representations

imagining – forming a mental image or concept; supposing

Usually the mistake is a lack of concentration rather than any semantic confusion.

The source of infection can be identified by ~~imagining~~ (**imaging**) *such as ultrasound or CT scanning.*

impair/impairment

impair – verb

impairment – noun

When referring to what the patients have, a noun will always be required not a verb.

The exclusion criteria included patients with renal or hepatic ~~impair~~ (**impairment**) *and those with...*

imply/infer

imply verb – to indicate or suggest without actually being stated

infer verb – to derive or conclude based on reasoning or evidence

These two verbs can be difficult to determine. Although on the surface they represent similar actions, their meanings are quite marked. Use 'infer' when you or someone comes to a conclusion about something based on the evidence available; use 'imply' to suggest an opinion or make an indirect statement that allows the reader to evaluate its value.

*The patient is able to ~~imply~~ (**infer**) that this is only temporary from the information provided.*

*The findings ~~infer~~ (**imply**) that the best course of treatment would be the former.*

Imply can also be used for when the writer does not actually believe it to be true.

*This **implies** that the staff could cope with the increase in administrative duties, which is highly unlikely.*

in detail

'details' is the plural form of the noun 'detail'.

*The key **details** of this trial can be found in the Appendix.*

'In (more) detail' is a fixed phrase meaning 'thoroughly'.

Do not use it as a plural.

*The findings will be discussed ~~in details~~ (**in detail**) in the next section.*

indentify

Despite its popularity on Google, there is actually no such word as 'indentify'.

*We will now **identify** the key reasons for why these treatments failed.*

infective/infectious

There is some overlap with these two adjectives but, in general, infectious refers to the spread of an infection, i.e. having the ability to be passed on or transmitted to others, while infective refers to its cause, i.e. having the ability to cause an infection.

*The **infectious** category includes diseases where the **infective** pathogen is responsible for the...*

*The ~~infectious~~ (**infective**) material is often transmitted by direct contact.*

The most common term using the 'infective' form is infective endocarditis

inhibit/inhabit

inhibit – to restrain, repress or prevent

inhabit – to exist or dwell somewhere

Both verbs are commonly used in the medical sciences. If the error is not a typo but uncertainty about the two verbs then think of staying somewhere as being a habit and so inhabiting.

*Bifidobacterium adolescentis has been shown to ~~inhabit~~ (**inhibit**) harmful bacterial enzyme activity...*

*The organ is ~~inhibited~~ (**inhabited**) by a vast number of microorganisms...*

The adjective form is 'inhibitory'.

*Saffron may have an ~~inhibit~~ (**inhibitory**) effect on free radical chain reactions.*

injury/injure

injury – noun (plural injuries)

injure – verb

The only issue that writers seem to have with these two terms is when the plural noun is required as seen here:

*Ossification is also common following blast ~~injures~~ (**injuries**) and hip replacement...*

inpatient/impatient

inpatient – a patient admitted to a hospital and whose treatment requires that they stay overnight

impatient – easily irritated; restless

This is a quirky error encouraged by keyboard layout.

This is a common problem that affects as many as 1 in 15 ~~impatients~~ *(**inpatients**).*

*We also ensured that the subjects would not get **impatient** by providing them with…*

instance/instant

instance noun – a case or example; an occurrence

instant noun or adjective – a short space of time; quick, immediate

The similarity here is a problem even for native speakers. Instant is probably more likely to be employed as an adjective than a noun as in the second 'instance' below.

We observed one ~~instant~~ *(**instance**) of this in each group.*

There was an ~~instance~~ *(**instant**) reduction in tumour size…*

intake

The opposite of intake is not outtake. Use expenditure instead.

Both intake and ~~outtake~~ *(**expenditure**) should be balanced.*

Do not split the term into two words.

Most patients underestimated their ~~in take~~ *(**intake**).*

intervene/intervention

intervene – verb

intervention – noun

Make sure you are using the correct form.

We decided a surgical ~~intervene~~ *(**intervention**) was required.*

And that the spelling is correct.

They felt it necessary to ~~intevene~~ *(**intervene**) given the severity of the situation.*

invasive/evasive

invasive adjective – tending to spread, often harmfully

evasive adjective – avoiding commitment; imprecise

~~Evasive~~ (**Invasive**) *aspergillosis can also present as septicaemia…*

The definition and example of invasive above describe diseases. Another common use of invasive is to describe procedures that intrude on the person and involve instruments being inserted into the body or body cavities.

This is a more ~~evasive~~ (***invasive***) *method for when results prove inconclusive.*

The noun form is 'invasiveness' not 'invasion'.

it

'It' should not be continually relied on to refer to a previous subject because ambiguity can result; however, it is useful for avoiding repetition of the subject and acting as a general sentence starter.

'It' can be used in a general way where it does not refer to anything in particular but forms a general description or experience of what follows.

It *is important to use the programs the clinic provides.*

Sometimes writers use 'this' when there is no direct reference with the preceding sentence. This is where 'it' can be employed as a link.

…and the stats may be weak in some areas; therefore, ~~this~~ (***it***) *is essential for data integrity to be maintained.*

But when used in this general way, 'it' cannot represent a noun and that noun cannot then follow.

It is important the parameter in the proposed scheme.   ✗

The sentence must be rearranged and the pronoun deleted.

The parameter is important…   ✓

A common error is using the singular possessive pronoun form (its) for a plural subject.

Managers of mature healthcare organisations are known for ~~its~~ (***their***) *adaptability in these situations.*

keep/remain

remain verb – to continue to be; to be left; to stay there

keep verb – to hold or retain; to maintain

'remain' and 'keep' are similar in meaning and either can be used in this example:

*It is crucial for the patient to **keep/remain** calm when this occurs.*

But when the meaning relates to something that continues to be or continues to exist then use 'remain'.

*This can ~~keep~~ (**remain**) a problem for those with low blood pressure.*

*The rate will ~~keeps~~ (**remain**) elevated for a number of minutes.*

And when the meaning relates to maintaining or holding on to something use 'keep'.

*They need to ~~remain~~ (**keep**) their form safe to prove their attendance...*

lack

The verb and noun forms of lack are often misused. A common error is using 'of' with the verb.

*The field still ~~lacks of~~ (**lacks**) research examining this disorder.*

Most lack ~~of~~ a suitable support network to deal with the...

It is the noun form that often occurs with 'of'.

*There was a **lack of** motivation in many of the subjects.*

There is a tendency for the verb to be overlooked. Here is a typical example of a writer opting for the noun phrase.

*The high mortality rate for ovarian serous carcinoma largely remains undetectable early on and ~~lack of~~ (**lacks**) reliable markers to evaluate its progression.*

A distinction can be made with the similar verb 'to fail'.

lack verb – to be without

fail verb – to fall short in achieving something

*This still ~~lacks~~ (**fails**) to explain why they did not respond to the original supplement.*

Do not confuse fail with fall.

*This is ignored as it ~~fails~~ (**falls**) outside the range.*

lay/lie

lay verb – to put something/someone down

lie verb – to rest or recline

So if someone is putting something down it is lay and if someone is setting themselves down somewhere it is lie.

The two problems here are the past tense and past participle forms and the fact that the simple present of lay and the simple past of lie are the same word – lay.

lay – present (lay) past (laid) past participle (laid)

The participants then laid their monitors down on the floor and reassembled...

lie – present (lie) past (lay) past participle (lain)

They then lay down on the bed ready for the final stage of the study.

lesion

lesion – A general term for a wound or patch of altered or infected tissue

legion – a vast number

Mass legions *(**lesions**) such as thrombus can occur within the heart...*

But note the spelling of Legionnaires' disease and the bacterium *Legionella*.

life/live

life – noun

live – verb

*These are conditions that can occur during the ~~live~~ (**life**) of a person with a disability.*

Matters are further complicated as live is also an adjective that is spelled the same as the verb, but it is pronounced differently to the verb and actually sounds similar to the noun.

verb *(liv)*   **adjective** *(laiv)*   **noun** *(līf)*

Alive is an adjective with a similar meaning but appears after the term it is describing.

*Their policy is not to test on ~~alive~~ (**live**) animals.*

*The rats were kept **alive** until...*

Note also that 'lifetime' is one word.

lightheaded

lightheaded – adjective

Sometimes the wordy noun form is required.

*The patient was experiencing periodic ~~lightheaded~~ (**lightheadedness**) and had a history of...*

loss/lose

'lose' is the verb and 'loss' is the noun

This was largely responsible for their ~~lose~~ *(**loss**) of balance.*

The impact was apparent on the data ~~loses~~ *(**loss**) rate.*

The plural noun is 'losses'.

This was a direct result of the ~~loses~~ *(**losses**) made by the clinic in the previous year.*

When the verb is required be careful not to use the unrelated adjective 'loose'.

In this case they may ~~loose~~ *(**lose**) sensation in their fingers or toes.*

This appears next to the ~~lose~~ *(**loose**) fibrous tissue.*

malignant/malignancy

malignant – adjective

malignancy – noun

When errors occur they are usually where the noun form has mistakenly been used as the adjective.

They carried out action research on improving end-of-life care to residents with a non-~~malignancy~~ *(**malignant**) disease.*

median/medial

medial adjective – relating to the middle; towards the middle

median noun – the middle

Median is used in 'median plane', the midline of the body and the 'median nerve' in the upper limb. It is also a statistical term often used for age, height, weight or survival rates.

*The **median** age at diagnosis is 65 years.*

Parts of the body with medial in their name include

medial malleolus   *medial meniscus*

medial lemniscus   *medial temporal lobe*

mobility/motility

Mobility is a general term for movement and is usually applied to things that are able to move but not necessarily on their own. Motility relates to something that can move by itself, i.e. active or spontaneous movement. Therefore we often refer to gut and sperm motility and joint mobility.

*Reduced gut ~~mobility~~ (**motility**) can lead to longer transit time and chronic constipation.*

morbidity/mortality

Morbidity refers to the health of a population, specifically the prevalence of disease.

Mortality refers to the number of deaths in a population.

*They looked at the leading causes of **morbidity** in week 16.*

*Morgan (2004) used data from a mixed-methods, cohort study to describe the patterns of **mortality**...*

So the morbidity rate looks at the incidence of a disease across a population and the mortality rate is the incidence of death in a population.

Comorbidity is the presence of additional disorders alongside a main disorder.

~~co-morbidity~~

obstruct/obstruction

obstruct – verb

obstruction – noun

obstructive – adjective

Take note of the endings of the three terms and be aware that the adjective form is likely to be part of a medical condition or process, not the verb or noun.

*The most common condition from the group was chronic ~~obstruction~~ (**obstructive**) pulmonary disease.*

*New vessels are accompanied by an ~~obstruct~~ (**obstruction**) at the drainage angle which creates...*

on average

Do not use 'averagely' to mean usually or typically. Use 'on average' instead.

*A meta-analysis suggested that it takes ~~averagely~~ (**on average**) three weeks for intrinsic motivation to be undermined...*

Also look out for ~~in average~~

overweight and obesity

Those not involved in the medical sciences would be surprised to find overweight being used as a noun in the following way:

*Since then, the prevalence of **overweight** and obesity has increased sharply in the country...*

Nevertheless, it is common in medical papers to use overweight in this way. Its use as a noun is also seen when referring to the collective group as one entity.

*Testing has shown that it reduces body weight in **the overweight** by...*

Overweight can be an adjective as well.

*They assessed twenty high quality studies that contained around 12,000 **overweight** or obese individuals.*

Obesity on the other hand cannot be used as an adjective. The adjective form is obese.

*A person with a BMI over 30 kg/m² is considered ~~obesity~~ (**obese**).*

Likewise, obese cannot be used as a noun.

*However, the cut-off point for those with ~~obese~~ (**obesity**) should be much lower...*

palpation/palpitation

palpate – verb to examine by touch

palpitate – verb to pulsate rapidly

These two are often mixed up. The nouns forms are palpation and palpitation.

Painless nodules should also be ~~palpitated~~ (palpated).

The patient was experiencing frequent ~~palpations~~ (palpitations).

periodic/periodical

period – noun

periodic – adjective

periodical – noun/adjective

periodically – adverb

Use 'periodic' for the adjective form as 'periodical' is used primarily as a noun for something that is published periodically.

Once diagnosed patients require ~~periodical~~ (periodic) assessment to ensure that...

predispose

predispose verb – to be more likely to behave in a particular way or be affected by a particular condition

This is apparent in genetically predisposed individuals who would...

The noun form is predisposition

Genetic predisposition and environmental influences are key contributors...

'Dispostion' relates more to character or general temperament.

An aggressive disposition will likely exacerbate these tension headaches...

present/refer

In the medical sciences a patient appearing for medical treatment may be said to 'present'. The sentence could simply describe the appearance of the patient in front of the medical professional.

*Patients rarely **present** to the doctor with a single surgical issue but in fact...*

'Present' can also be used to reveal what the patient is suffering from. When the condition or symptom is revealed they 'present with'.

*Subjects **presented with** painful swelling of the legs and...*

*Oesophageal cancer patients most often **present with** dysphagia...*

It can also be used as an adjective.

*This will often occur as the **presenting** feature in elderly patients.*

However, many journals and schools avoid 'presented' and instead advise their writers to use 'sought treatment for' or 'were suffering from'.

'refer' has many uses, one of which is when a patient is sent elsewhere for treatment.

*The patient was **referred** to a specialist clinic...*

Another is related to localised pain or pain felt somewhere other than the primary site.

*In this instance the pain was **referred** from the diaphragm.*

Note the following error:

*When a patient ~~refers with~~ (**presents with**) these symptoms they should be...*

The writer can just as easily use 'has'.

*When a patient **has** these symptoms they should be...*

prevalence/prevalent

prevalence – noun

prevalent – adjective

*...Streptococcus spp. was more ~~prevalence~~ (**prevalent**) in colorectal adenoma patients.*

*The ~~prevalent~~ (**prevalence**) of functional constipation has been studied...*

Prevalence is used with a percentage or a ratio. It cannot be measured by just a number.

The third city had a lower obesity prevalence at around 400,000.   ✗

The third city had a lower obesity prevalence at around 11%.   ✓

principal/principle

principal adjective – first or highest in rank; chief

principle noun – a rule of action or general law

These terms are pronounced the same but have very different meanings. When in doubt think of *principal*ity, where a high 'chief' or the 'first' prince might live.

*The basic **principle** of the TEN test is to control for...*

*The flavones were the **principal** components and the potential of individual compounds was assessed using...*

*In ~~principal~~ (**principle**), this should be a simple task...*

prospective

prospective – expected or likely to happen in the future

Prospective is often employed to refer to studies or students.

Prospective studies follow a population from an initial condition to a stage in the future.

*This was further confirmed by a two year longitudinal **prospective** study...*

Prospective students refer to individuals who may attend an institution or enroll on a course in the future.

Sometimes the term is confused with 'perspective', which refers to someone's point of view or attitude about something.

*This has been validated in research utilising ~~perspective~~ (**prospective**), randomized, and crossover trials.*

prosthesis

Prosthesis is a noun with two meanings. It can refer to an artificial device substituting for a body part or the process of replacing a missing body part with a device. Note the article use for each:

*Amputees were asked to use **a prosthesis** from the selection provided for at least three weeks.*

*An early paper (12) looking at oesophageal replacement with **prosthesis** devised a combination of...*

A person who specialises in the area of prosthetics is a prosthetist. The adjective form is prosthetic. Compare the noun and adjective endings.

noun – prosthe**sis**   ~~prosthetis~~
adjective – prosthe**tic** ~~prosthesic~~

rationale

rational adjective – reasonable, sensible

rationale noun – the main reason accounting for something

Most of the time the writer means 'rationale'.

*The ~~rational~~ (**rationale**) for using this intensity was to maximise the sensitivity in order to detect differences between the two groups.*

recur/reoccur

There is a subtle difference between these two verbs. Something recurring happens at regular intervals or just repeatedly. Something reoccurring happens again but maybe just once. These examples will illustrate the distinction.

*Oral cancer can **reoccur** yet studies up to now seem to have taken only a limited number of factors into account…* (occurring again)

*The malady often **recurs** three or more times a year, and can last a number of weeks.* (repeatedly occurring)

recur has a noun and adjective form. Note the double 'r' in the middle.

recurrence – noun   recurrent – adjective

Given its principal meaning of happening just once more, the adjective form of reoccur (reoccurrent) is used much less than recurrent; the noun 'reoccurrence' is frequently adopted though. Again note the spelling.

*The **reoccurrence** of gout has been linked to levels of humidity…*

Spelling the present participle also seems to be an issue.

~~reoccuring~~   ~~reocurring~~

reduce/reduction

reduce – verb

reduction – noun

'reduce' cannot be used as a noun.

UVA does result in a significant ~~reduce~~ (reduction) in enzymatic activity...

There can be an increase and a decrease but not a reduce – It is a reduction.

reflex/reflux

reflex – automatic action or movement of the body in response to something

reflux – to flow back or return, e.g. contents from the stomach back up to the oesophagus

These two are similar in that they both relate to an action of the body. The process of reflux is specific whereas a reflex has a more versatile use and can be used figuratively as well as for a spontaneous movement of the body.

This has also been attributed to bile salts due to ~~reflex~~ (reflux).

We were looking for parameters that would minimise the involvement of middle ear muscle ~~refluxes~~ (reflexes).

regime/regimen

'regimen' has always been the preferred noun to denote a regulated course relating to treatment, diet, exercise or lifestyle in general. The primary use of 'regime' is in political matters but it can be employed in the same way as 'regimen' for a systematic and regulated approach to something.

If a distinction must be made then perhaps 'regime' is better suited in a general sense and as a plural, and 'regimen' for a specific instance and as a singular noun.

*The exercise **regimen** will be based on the physical condition of the individual participant.*

*The next stage will be to design some exercise **regimes** to assess the two groups.*

relief/relieve

relief – noun

relieve – verb

*It has also been suggested that these alternative medicines offer partial symptom ~~relieve~~ (**relief**) at best.*

*Topical capsaicin has been shown to ~~relief~~ (**relieve**) both pruritus and pain...*

The noun is often used with 'from'.

*~~Relieve~~ (**Relief**) from bloating was assessed using...*

In medicine the verb form usually takes 'by'.

*In the majority of cases it is **relieved by** rest.*

remain/stay

There is little semantic difference between the two terms but there are some expressions where one or the other is employed. Here are some instances of 'remain'.

The role of these drugs remains unclear.

This remains the preferred choice...

Some will remain even after prolonged treatment.

'Stay' works well in more informal circumstances.

The slogan 'Stay fit, stay happy' appeared on the leaflets that were distributed to...

Did you stay there longer than three weeks?

'Stay' can also be a noun.

*This would require a short **stay** at the hospital, at least until...*

respectively

'Respectively' is used for parallel lists to inform the reader that a second list is in the same order as a previous list of things. It is employed to avoid repetition by not having to write out all the elements again.

It is not required if an earlier reference has not been made.

There is a brief consultation and a thorough examination ~~respectively~~.

This following list of numbers does not refer to any previous list of items, so 'respectively' is not needed.

The levels chosen were 0.2, 0.4, 0.6 and 0.8 ~~respectively~~.

Here 'respectively' can be used because there is an earlier reference:

*The cooked, cooled and reheated potatoes produced 4.6%, 20.3% and 4.1% of resistant starch **respectively.***

respond/response

respond – verb

response – noun

Writers sometimes discuss patients 'responsing' to treatment or the 'respond' rates to their surveys; these mistakes need to be addressed.

*Group three should ~~response~~ (**respond**) to the treatment quicker than Group two.*

*The **response** rate was better than expected…*

*Patients producing a good immune ~~respond~~ (**response**) would be more likely to…*

result/occur

occur verb – to happen; to take place

result verb – to end up being; to be the outcome of

*This sensation ~~results~~ (**occurs**) at different times of the day...*

*The difference in the size of the two regions ~~occuring~~ (**results**) in an adjustment being made to...*

Result is less flexible in terms of prepositional use and is found only with 'from' and 'in'.

result from – to be caused by

result in – to cause a situation to happen

*This impairment **results from** an infection of the inner ear...*

'Result' is also erroneously used instead of 'test'.

*Our other patient also ~~resulted~~ (**tested**) positive for this.*

resume/resumption

resume – verb

resumption – noun

Resumption is rarely misidentified as a verb but resume is turned into a noun by some writers.

*The ~~resume~~ (**resumption**) of this treatment may lead to a return of the complaint.*

*We **resumed** interviews with the patients a week later...*

reveal/exhibit

reveal – to make known

exhibit – to display, show or present

There is some overlap but generally patients exhibit signs and symptoms, and tests and trials reveal the nature of the problem.

*This ~~exhibits~~ (**reveals**) the unexpected role that plumbagin plays in the...*

*As the patient was **exhibiting** signs of stress during the consultation, we decided to...*

reverse/reversal

Reverse can be a noun, adjective or verb.

This trend was reversed less than two weeks later.

Reversal is a noun and is the correct option in these examples.

*The ~~reverse~~ (**reversal**) of this measure leads to a much faster recovery.*

*This was not the only study to report a ~~reverse~~ (**reversal**) in the lipid profile levels.*

Also note the following error:

*Patients in the placebo group received the treatments in ~~reversed~~ (**reverse**) order.*

rigour/rigorous

rigour as a noun and rigorous as an adjective relate to taking care and being thorough. In American English the noun is spelled rigor. It has the alternative meaning of onset of a fever and is also used for stiffness as in the condition *rigor mortis*.

The noun is uncountable so has no plural form. The following error is common:

*~~Rigours~~ (**Rigorous**) testing is necessary for the identification of...*

rise/raise

rise   verb – to increase

          noun – an increase; an act of rising

raise verb – to lift up; to elevate

          noun – an increase in

          amount (especially salary)

'Raise' as a verb always has an object linked to it.

*Our modification was able to **raise** the concentration in over half of the samples.*

'Rise' as a verb is used on its own and does not require a direct object.

*The levels will **rise** again if the dosage is not adhered to.*

As a rule we 'raise' something but something 'rises'.

'Rise' is an irregular verb.

Present simple:

I/we/they rise

It/he/she rises

Present participle: rising

Past participle: risen

Past simple: rose

Often the wrong verb or verb form is selected.

*In 2011, the number of companies producing these drugs ~~raised~~ (**rose**) to six.*

*The ~~rose~~ (**rise**) and fall in temperature was noted down for twelve hours.*

*This also ~~rose~~ (**raised**) the white cell count and the sedimentation rate.*

Also, 'arise' meaning to emerge or become apparent is confused with both of these terms.

*This ~~arises~~ (**raises**) the possibility of infection considerably.*

same/similar

same – identical

similar – having a likeness or resemblance

*These figures were the ~~similar~~ (**same**) as the previous ones.*

*or/ These figures were **similar** to the previous ones.*

*A ~~same~~ (**similar**) trend has been reported in Sweden (12).*

*or/ The **same** trend has been reported in Sweden (12).*

'Same' is always used with a definite article.

Mistakes usually occur when the writer states that something is identical (*same*) when they actually want to say there are just some things in common (*similar*).

Also, do not write '~~almost similar~~'.

Use 'similar' or 'almost the same'.

severe/severity

severe – adjective

severity – noun

Avoid using 'severeness' for the noun.

*This depends on the ~~severeness~~ (**severity**) of the inflammation.*

*If there is ~~severity~~ (**severe**) and constant pain then the first option is more appropriate.*

*A number of ~~severity~~ (**severe**) cases have been reported that involved...*

simulate/stimulate

simulate – to create a likeness or a model of a system or situation

stimulate – to excite or rouse to action

That second letter makes all the difference.

*These models were not able to effectively ~~stimulate~~ (**simulate**) the observed in vivo profile.*

*As a result, the auditory nerve fibres will not respond when ~~simulated~~ (**stimulated**).*

The noun forms are simulation and stimulation. The former is a countable noun and the latter more commonly used in an uncountable way.

*Repeated ~~stimulations~~ (**stimulation**) of these zones can lead to nausea and vomiting.*

sit/seat

seat noun – something on which a person can sit

seating noun – the assigning of seats; the layout of a venue

Mistakes occur when a form of the verb 'to sit' is desired.

*Sedentary behaviour such as ~~seating~~ (**sitting**) or lying is a primary cause of...*

*'I am in pain even if I ~~seat~~ (**sit**) down'.*

Seat as a verb is uncommon and usually refers to the capacity of a venue.

strain/stain

strain   verb – to stretch or exert muscles or nerves; to overexert one-self; to filter liquid

noun – pressure or stress on one's body; organisms of the same species having distinctive characteristics, such as a variety of bacterium; lines of ancestry

stain   verb – to leave a mark or change the colour of something; to treat specimens for microscopic study

noun – a mark on the surface of the skin; a substance used to colour tissue and cells, the resulting sample or test

This is more often a typo than a lack of understanding and it is usually the noun instances that lead to the mistakes.

*Mice from each ~~stain~~ (**strain**) were then injected with CTX…*

*The second exercise was identified as placing too much **strain** on the body.*

*This was used to confirm the type of saliva ~~strain~~ (**stain**) and then determine the age of it.*

success/successful

success – noun

successful – adjective

The noun and the adjective are sometimes mixed up.

*Overall, the treatment was deemed a ~~successful~~ (**success**).*

*They also achieved a ~~success~~ (**successful**) outcome but with a smaller number.*

Note also the verb 'to succeed'.

*…however, the ~~succeed~~ (**success**) rates are fairly low.*

*The report looked at the rising number of students failing to **succeed** at medical school.*

survive/survival

survive – verb

survival – noun

*We also revealed that it played a major role in cell ~~survive~~ **(survival)** and differentiation.*

*Around 80% of patients respond to treatment and ~~survival~~ **(survive)** after an initial episode.*

Survival can also be used as an adjective and is often seen paired with rate.

*The 5-year **survival** rate is close to 80%.*

systemic/systematic

systemic	adjective – relating to or affecting the entire body or a particular body system (such as the digestive system)
systematic	adjective – in an organised manner or according to a system

Although 'systemic' can also be used to describe a system-based approach, it is sensible to use 'systematic' for this purpose given the well-used medical definition of systemic above.

*These types of studies can help to understand the local and **systemic** biological activities of the class...*

*There have been a number of **systematic** reviews and meta-analyses of the effectiveness of probiotics...*

Check your spelling: ~~sistemic~~

threat/threaten

threat – noun

threaten – verb

Using the base form of the verb (*threaten*) as the noun is an extremely common mistake.

*This particular strain has proven to be less of a ~~threaten~~ (**threat**) than previously thought.*

*Behaviour change occurred because of the perceived **threat** from their continued unhealthy lifestyle.*

'life-threatening' is an associated adjective.

*Leaving the conditions untreated is potentially **life-threatening**.*

tolerate/tolerance

tolerate – verb

tolerance – noun

tolerant – adjective

Keep an eye on these three similar forms:

*We measured their perceived ~~tolerant~~ (**tolerance**) to the following:*

*The soft tissue is not designed to **tolerate** forces of this nature.*

***Tolerance** to this is naturally much higher in humans than in rats.*

Intolerance and intolerant are the negative forms.

topical/tropical

topical   adjective – applied to the surface of a local or specific area of the body

tropical   adjective – pertaining to the tropics and usually the insects/diseases associated with those areas

Here is another pair of adjectives distinct in meaning but similar in form. Two typical sentences in which they occur are

*Certain **topical** emollients can be applied to reduce the dryness...*

*Their work primarily took place in **tropical** settings and involved testing...*

track/tract

track – a mark or indentation; a path or route

tract – an elongated set of organs arranged in series and providing a particular function; a set of axons grouped together to form a pathway

Common tracts in the human body include

digestive tract   intestinal tract

respiratory tract   urinal tract   uveal tract

The lateral lemniscus is a ~~track~~ *(**tract**) of axons carrying sound to the inferior colliculus in the auditory midbrain.*

Subsequently, they studied the association of symptoms in the upper and lower gastrointestinal ~~track~~ *(**tract**).*

There is also a verb form.

*The device allows us to **track** the progress of the disease…*

trial/trail

Although more often than not a typo, this is nevertheless prolific. A 'trial' is an experimental action. A 'trail' is a track or a path.

They carried out a randomised clinical ~~trail~~ *(**trial**).*

During the second ~~trail~~ *(**trial**) the intake was tracked.*

trophic/tropic

trophic – stimulating, nourishing; growth

tropic – turning or changing; having an influence on

Check your use of these suffixes. Use –tropic for change or influence and –trophic for growth.

hepatotropic – having a specific effect or influence on the liver

neurotropic – having a specific effect or influence on the nervous system

hypertrophic – exhibiting an increase in size or volume (of an organ or tissue)

atrophic – wasting away of the body or part of the body

unstable

The adjective form for describing something that is not stable is 'unstable' not 'instable'.

*They also had an ~~instable~~ (**unstable**) diet profile.*

Confusion probably stems from the term 'instability'. This is the noun form.

*This will contribute to genetic ~~unstability~~ (**instability**).*

upregulation

upregulation – noun

upregulate – verb

These terms are one word.

*They reported increased expression of MRF4 mRNA correlating with ~~up regulation~~ (**upregulation**) of COX-2…*

This also applies to downregulation/downregulate.

versus/vs.

The term should always be written in full when it is part of the main text.

*The sample was randomised to receive low dose (1.6 mg/defect) **versus** carrier control…*

vs. can be used for results in bracketed text. A full stop must follow this abbreviated form.

*(1744.3, IQR 1702.4 **vs.** 3571.4, IQR 4208.5)*

v is used for legal cases.

*Fox **v** General Medical Council [1960]*

void

void   verb – to discharge waste from the body

noun – an empty space

adjective – unoccupied

Make sure not to confuse any of these with 'avoid'.

Obstruction causes severe discomfort and a desire to ~~avoid~~ *(**void**) urine.*

*Water is held on the hydrophilic sites of the fibre itself or within **void** spaces in the molecular structure.*

SECTION V

Aftercare

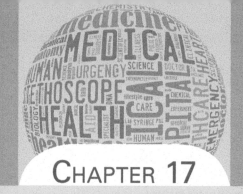

Chapter 17

Aftercare

Exercises

The following exercises target the mistakes that you and your colleagues are making when writing in English. Identify and correct these and you will be well on your way to achieving error-free English.

Remedies for nouns and articles

A1 How many sentences are incorrect?

Statistical analysis was carried out in three stages.

Morgan also analyses the reasons why the levels remained so low.

It would also be useful if analyse of the data was expanded to peripheral sites.

A2 How many of these singular to plural transformations are wrong?

cortex	→	cortices
hypothesis	→	hypothesise
prosthesis	→	prosthetics
varix	→	varices

A3 How many of these usually uncountable nouns can also be used in a countable way?

equipment   support   staff   training

A4 A or an?

_____ *European case study will also be adopted.*

We decided to take _____ *average score instead.*

The patient was advised to go for _____ *ECG.*

A5 Do any of these need a definite article?

This can be done on _____ *regular basis.*

It appears _____ *aim of their project was to...*

The treatment tends to work at _____ *first and then...*

Then _____ *group was transfected with COX-2...*

Of course, _____ *communication is important at this point...*

A6 How many noun and article errors has the writer made?

In this studies, the audiological measures were used to investigate auditory dysfunction in tinnitus patients with the normal hearing. The general aim was to investigate the peripheral source of tinnitus in patients with normal hearing so as to provide an objective evidences for guiding their rehabilitative management and treatment.

Remedies for verbs

B1 'was' 'been', 'has been' or 'being'?

Cells were cultured for 48 h before _____ *co-transfected...*

Within 120 minutes of _____ *consumed it enters the colon...*

This definition _____ *widely adopted by clinicians.*

At the time the infection _____ *virtually unknown.*

B2 Singular or plural verb?

Information on the various reasons is/are *required before...*

Sufficient evidence has/have *been found to show that...*

The expression in different histopathological subgroups was/were *highly correlated.*

Active or sham stimulation was/were *employed for...*

B3 Which form of these troublesome verbs should be used?

This remains the most important risk factor for patients undergo/undergoing/underwent *surgery.*

However, four patients withdraw/withdrawn/withdrew *from the study due to...*

For those seek/sought/seeking *medical help there are a few procedures that...*

B4 Can you identify four modal errors?

Recent studies suggest that this may even contributes to the increase. In the next section we would evaluate the various methods and hypothesise that the lack of a consensus might because of the way results are reported, while a final discussion should to resolve the issues stated earlier.

Remedies for adjectives and adverbs

C1 Noun or adjective ending?

There was a considerable differen _____ *between the two...*

These spores are also resistan _____ *to boiling and...*

One patient had been suffering from a persisten _____ *cough.*

They varied in importan _____ *as well as structure.*

C2 fewer or less?

_____ *than six is considered a satisfactory result.*

They had significantly _____ *illness episodes.*

Those experiencing _____ pain were placed in group B.

One criticism was that they provided _____ data.

C3 Which ones in each row can take a singular verb?

any   enough little   _____

many   some   those   _____

another either   other   _____

Remedies for prepositions

D1 on, in or at?

Most of the respondents worked _____ the hospital.

This took place _____ 16th May.

It was then placed _____ a 2 L beaker and incubated _____ 37°C

It tends to form _____ the hands and feet.

D2 What preposition should follow?

This is primarily caused _____ a lack of vitamin D.

The patient's pain was confined _____ the lower back

What impact does this have _____ nurses and carers?

These services need to be more responsive _____ the needs of the patients.

Remedies for all complaints

E1 Cross out the unnecessary words. Can you reduce this passage to under 50 words?

The systematic approach usually starts by distinguishing objective tinnitus (OT) and subjective tinnitus (ST). Moreover, it is very crucial to differentiate objective tinnitus from subjective tinnitus because failure to make a distinction may lead to management errors, while diagnostic issues will continue to remain as well (12). In addition to the above, ultimately this step is important for identifying any potential treatable disorders. These are listed in Table 2.1.

E2 Can you make the right selections?

In a/an/the *multicentre study setting seven health clinics provided ten subjects each, of varying age and mixed gender. Therefore* 70/seventy *subjects were recruited* totally/in total/averagely *(25 men, 45 women, mean age 39.2 years, range 22–69). In order to evaluate the intra-individual variation a repeated* exam/examine/examination *was carried out on ten subjects at two different centres....in paper III ten healthy* man/men/male's *were recruited and studied in a randomised cross-over fashion* at/in/on *two occasions, two weeks apart...we* can/will/would *review this next along with the author's previous paper on bile acid malabsorption and* its/it's *correlation with bowel transit.*

E3 How many mistakes are in this abstract?

Pulmonary gas exchange was studied in 12 patients with spontaneous pneumothorax by measuring the partial pressure of oxygen and carbon doxide in arterially blood and expired gas when breathing air and 100% of oxygen. There were a positive correlated between the size of the anatomical shunt and the extend of the pneumothorax as measured bye the chest radiograph. Calculations indicated that the fall on arterial oxygen tension when breathing air could be full accounted for by the increased anatomical shunt. Observations suggested that active vasoconstriction in poor ventilated regions may have occured to a slight or moderate degree in four out of eight patience.

E4 Can you amend the questions?

How the service can be improved?

How would you describe their quality of life in nursing home?

How they view the role of the pharmacist?

What is important to the patient daily life in the nursing home?

What should make their quality of life better?

They have access to any other services?

E5 Can you capture all the spelling and punctuation errors?

The TEN test has been used, to investigate the presense of dead regions in patient's with tinnitus. In a study by Weisz at al. (2006), the TEN (SPL) test and tinitus spectrum-test were carried out on (11 tinnitus patients) who self-reported having normal hearing and subjective cronic tinnitus. The study found that, the reference freqeuncy threshold showed a strong increase (mean; 8.4; SE = 1.5). Whereas thresholds at other frequencys were at a low level.

Answers

A1

One. *It would also be useful if* ~~analyse~~ *(**analysis**) of the data was expanded to peripheral sites.*

A2

hypothesis ⟶ ~~hypothesise~~ (***hypotheses***)

prosthesis ⟶ ~~prosthetics~~ (***prostheses***)

A3

None of them.

A4

A European case study will also be adopted.

*We decided to take **an** average score instead.*

*The patient was advised to go for **an** ECG.*

A5

*It appears **the** aim of their project was to...*

*Then **the** group was transfected with COX-2...*

A6

In this ~~studies~~ *(**study**),* ~~the~~ *audiological measures were used to investigate auditory dysfunction in tinnitus patients with* ~~the~~ *normal hearing. The general aim was to investigate the peripheral source of tinnitus in patients with normal hearing so as to provide* ~~an~~ *objective* ~~evidences~~ *(**evidence**) for guiding their rehabilitative management and treatment.*

B1

*Cells were cultured for 48 h before **being** co-transfected...*

*Within 120 minutes of **being** consumed it enters the colon...*

*This definition **has been** widely adopted by clinicians.*

*At the time the infection **was** virtually unknown.*

B2

*Information on the various reasons **is** required before...*

*Sufficient evidence **has** been found to show that...*

*The expression in different histopathological subgroups **was** highly correlated.*

*Active or sham stimulation **was** employed for...*

B3

*This remains the most important risk factor for patients **undergoing** surgery.*

*However, four patients **withdrew** from the study due to...*

*For those **seeking** medical help there are a few procedures that...*

B4

*Recent studies suggest that this may even contributes to the increase. In the next section we ~~would~~ (**will**) evaluate the various methods and hypothesise that the lack of a consensus might (**be**) because of the way results are reported, while a final discussion should ~~to~~ resolve the issues stated earlier.*

C1

*There was a considerable **difference** between the two...*

*These spores are also **resistant** to boiling and...*

*One patient had been suffering from a **persistent** cough.*

*They varied in **importance** as well as structure.*

C2

***Fewer** than six is considered a satisfactory result.*

*They had significantly **fewer** illness episodes.*

*Those experiencing **less** pain were placed in group B.*

*One criticism was that they provided **less** data.*

C3

any	*enough*	*little*
many	*some*	*those*
another	*either*	*other*

D1

Most of the respondents worked at the hospital.

This took place on 16th May.

It was then placed in a 2 L beaker and incubated at 37°C.

It tends to form on the hands and feet.

D2

This is primarily caused by a lack of vitamin D.

The patient's pain was confined to the lower back.

What impact does this have on nurses and carers?

These services need to be more responsive to the needs of the patients.

E1

The systematic approach usually starts by distinguishing objective tinnitus (OT) and subjective tinnitus (ST). It is crucial to differentiate OT from ST because failure to make a distinction may lead to management errors and diagnostic issues (12). This step is important for identifying any treatable disorders (Table 2.1).

E2

In a multicentre study setting seven health clinics provided ten subjects each, of varying age and mixed gender. Therefore 70 subjects were recruited in total (25 men, 45 women, mean age 39.2 years, range 22–69). In order to evaluate the intra-individual variation a repeated examination was carried out on ten subjects at two different centres.... in paper III ten healthy men were recruited and studied in a randomised cross-over fashion on two occasions, two weeks apart...we will review this next along with the author's previous paper on bile acid malabsorption and its correlation with bowel transit.

E3

(Twelve errors - corrections in bold) *Pulmonary gas exchange was studied in 12 patients with spontaneous pneumothorax by measuring the partial pressure of oxygen and carbon **dioxide** in **arterial** blood and expired gas when breathing air and **100% oxygen**. There **was** a positive **correlation** between the size of the anatomical shunt and the **extent** of the pneumothorax as measured **by** the chest radiograph. Calculations indicated that the fall **in** arterial oxygen tension when breathing air could be **fully** accounted for by the increased anatomical shunt. Observations suggested that active vaso - constriction in **poorly** ventilated regions may have **occurred** to a slight or moderate degree in four out of eight **patients**.*

E4

How can the service be improved?

How would you describe their quality of life in the nursing home?

How do they view the role of the pharmacist?

What is important to the patient's daily life in the nursing home?

What would/could make their quality of life better?

Do they have access to any other services?

E5

*The TEN test has been **used to** investigate the **presence** of dead regions in **patients** with tinnitus. In a study by Weisz **et** al. (2006), the TEN (SPL) test and **tinnitus spectrum test** were carried out on **11 tinnitus patients** who self-reported having normal hearing and subjective **chronic** tinnitus. The study found **that** the reference **frequency** threshold showed a strong increase (mean; 8.4; SE = 1.5)**, whereas** thresholds at other **frequencies** were at a low level.*

Index